FINAL FRCA PRACTICE PAPERS

FINAL FRCA PRACTICE PAPERS

Tim Isitt MRCP FRCA
Senior Registrar in Anaesthetics,
The Middlesex Hospital, London.

Sarah Chieveley-Williams MRCP FRCA
Senior Registrar in Anaesthetics,
The Middlesex Hospital, London.

PASTEST
Dedicated to your success

Egerton Court
Parkgate Estate
Knutsford
Cheshire WA16 8DX

First published 1998
Reprinted 1999
ISBN 1 901198 03 0

A catalogue record for this book is available from the British Library.

Typeset by Breeze Ltd, Manchester.
Printed by MPG Books Limited, Bodmin.

CONTENTS

FOREWORD

The increase in factual knowledge needed to keep up with developments in anaesthesia and intensive care means that a student's time must be directed towards learning the essentials of the subject and the all important techniques required to answer multiple choice question and short answer question papers.

Many MCQ books have been produced which have verbose and ambiguous stems to their questions and leave the candidate with doubtful choices. Poorly designed MCQs do not simulate the Fellowship examination and are not useful preparation for the examination candidate. The MCQs in this book are concise, precise and give a wide coverage of the breadth and depth of modern anaesthesia.

The new final FRCA examination incorporates short answer questions and clinical/clinical science vivas. The absence of traditional essay questions gives candidates little opportunity to plan answers and show prioritisation and judgement. In my view, the short answer and structural questions, like the MCQs, test rapid recall of detailed factual information.

Many candidates will only score good marks in the examination when they have acquired, through practice questions, the skills required to complete a full short answer paper in the limited time available in the examination.

This book combines the methods that students must learn in order to develop good examination technique with the educational role of a good textbook. The information provided is so up-to-date and clinically relevant that both teachers and students will find it a worthwhile purchase.

Ronald Greenbaum
Consultant, Department of Anaesthesia
The Middlesex and University College Hospitals
London

INTRODUCTION

The new Final Examination for the Diploma of Fellow of the Royal College of Anaesthetists was introduced in November 1996. Details of the entry requirements for the examination and a full syllabus are available from **The Royal College of Anaesthetists, 48-49 Russell Square, London WC1B 4JY**.

To be eligible to take the examination, a candidate must

- be registered with the General Medical Council
- be working in a recognised Specialist Registrar training post
- have completed at least 30 months' training in anaesthetics.

The Final Examination consists of a written Short Answer paper, an MCQ paper and two Vivas. All four parts of the examination are close-marked.

The scoring scheme for each paper is as follows:

0 A bad fail
1 A fail
1+ A bare fail
2 A pass
2+ A good pass

In order to pass the written papers and progress to the vivas, a candidate must score at least 2 for one of the written papers and at least 1+ for the other written paper. A score of 1 or below in any section of the examination will automatically mean a fail overall, no matter how high the scores in other parts of the examination.

The Short Answer Paper

This normally takes place during the morning of the examination; the MCQ paper takes place in the afternoon. Three hours are allowed for the candidate to complete two papers, each containing six questions. All twelve questions are compulsory and candidates who do not answer every question will fail the exam.

The questions will tend to follow the following format:

1. Paediatric
2. Neurosurgical
3. Obstetric
4. Cardiothoracic
5. Emergency/Trauma

6. Pain (acute and chronic)
7. Intensive Care (without burns)
8. Intensive Care (with burns)
9. Clinical Measurement
10. Regional/Local Anaesthesia
11. Medicine/Surgery
12. Dental/Maxillofacial/ENT/Ophthalmology

The questions in this book follow a similar format. A specimen SAQ paper can be obtained from either College Tutors or directly from the Education Department at the Royal College of Anaesthetists.

The MCQ Paper
Three hours are allowed for the candidate to complete 90 multiple choice questions. The MCQs are negatively marked, therefore if you are very uncertain of an answer it is best not to guess at it. The approximate breakdown of the paper is as follows:

- 20 questions on medicine and surgery
- 20 questions on pain and anaesthesia
- 20 questions on intensive care
- 20 questions on pharmacology and physiology
- 10 questions on clinical measurement.

The Vivas
If you achieve an adequate score in the two written papers you will be invited to attend the vivas. These take place at the Royal College four to five weeks after the written examination. In any given viva session all candidates are asked the same questions.

Viva 1 - The Clinical Viva (50 minutes)
You are given 10 minutes to study some clinical data, usually a case history with biochemical and haematological test results, an ECG and a chest X-ray. You then spend 20 minutes discussing this material with an examiner. Finally you will spend another 20 minutes with a second examiner discussing several unrelated clinical scenarios.

Viva 2 (30 minutes)
This viva is intended to focus on intensive care, pain management and the application of basic sciences to these disciplines. There are two examiners and you will spend 15 minutes with each of them.

In the RCA Newsletter of July 1996, the Examinations Audit Working Party published an article on structured vivas with examples of the "ultimate" viva questions – questions which accurately discriminated between pass and fail candidates. The topics highlighted were:

- the anaesthetic management of a patient requiring thyroidectomy
- the problems associated with anaesthetising an intravenous drug user
- the effects of intermittent positive pressure ventilation
- analgesics.

It would therefore seem wise to consider these topics as part of your preparation for the vivas!

How To Use This Book

This book contains three complete SAQ papers, three MCQ papers and three mock vivas. All of the questions are designed to be very similar to those likely to be encountered in the examination. The book is arranged in the format of three complete mock examinations.

To derive the most benefit from this book we recommend that you work systematically through each complete paper under timed conditions (and do not be tempted to look at the answers). This will help you to develop your examination technique as well as highlighting your personal strengths and weaknesses in time for further study. The answers and explanations at the end of each examination include references to key journal articles for further reading.

There is no substitute for a sound knowledge base and no candidate can pass the examination without this. However, an understanding of the structure of the exam and plenty of practice on MCQs, SAQs and vivas will increase your chances of success.

Good luck!

Tim Isitt
Sarah Chieveley-Williams

ABBREVIATIONS

ADH	Antidiuretic hormone
APTT	Activated partial thromboplastin time
ARDS	Acute respiratory distress syndrome
ASD	Atrial septal defect
ATN	Acute tubular necrosis
CCF	Congestive cardiac failure
CO	Carbon monoxide
CPAP	Continuous positive airway pressure
CVP	Central venous pressure
DDAVP	Desmopressin
DIC	Disseminated intravascular coagulation
DVT	Deep vein thrombosis
EDRF	Endothelin derived relaxant factor
EMD	Electromechanical dissociation
ETT	Endotracheal tube
FFP	Fresh frozen plasma
FGF	Fresh gas flow
FRC	Functional residual capacity
GCS	Glasgow coma scale
GTN	Glyceryl trinitrate
HDU	High dependency unit
HELLP	Haemolysis, elevated liver function tests and low platelets
HOCM	Hypertrophic obstructive cardiomyopathy
HRT	Hormone replacement therapy
IAP	Intra-abdominal pressure
INF	International normalised ratio
IOP	Intraocular pressure
JVP	Jugular venous pressure
LVF	Left ventricular failure

MAOIs	Monoamine oxidase inhibitors
MAC	Minimum alveolar concentration
MCV	Mean corpuscular volume
MDMA	Ecstasy
MH	Malignant hyperpyrexia
N_2O	Nitrous oxide
NMDA	N-methyl-D-aspartate
NSAIDs	Non-steroidal anti-inflammatory drugs
OCP	Oral contraceptive pill
PAOP	Pulmonary artery occlusive pressure
PCA	Patient controlled analgesia
PDA	Patent ductus arteriosus
PDPH	Post dural puncture headache
PE	Pulmonary embolus
PEA	Pulseless electrical activity
PEEP	Positive end expiratory pressure
PEFR	Peak expiratory flow rate
PT	Prothrombin time
SIADH	Syndrome of inappropriate antidiuretic hormone
rTPA	Recombinant tissue plasminogen activator
TLCO	Carbon monoxide transfer factor
TPN	Total parenteral nutrition
TV	Tidal volume
VSD	Ventricular septal defect

RECOMMENDED READING LIST

There are many excellent textbooks on the market. Listed below are the books I found personally of great use for the Final FRCA examination.

A-Z of Anaesthesia: Yentis S, Hirsch N P and Smith G P, 2nd edition, Butterworth Heinemann 1995.

Clinical Textbook of Anaesthesia: Aitkinhead A R and Jones R M, Churchill Livingstone 1996.

Acute Medicine Algorithm: Singer M and Webb A, Oxford University Press 1994.

Essays and MCQs in Anaesthesia and Intensive Care: Murphy P M, Edward Arnold 1994.

Handbook of Clinical Anaesthesia: Goldstone J C and Pollard B J, Churchill Livingstone 1996.

Intensive Care: Hinds C J, 2nd edition, Ballière Tindall 1995.

Key Topics in Anaesthesia: Craft T and Upton P, 2nd edition, Bios 1995.

Numerous journals are available, listed below are some that I found very useful:

Anaesthesiology

British Journal of Anaesthesia - editorials and reviews are often very good

British Journal of Hospital Medicine

British Medical Journal

Current Anaesthesia and Critical Care

Current Opinions in Anaesthesiology

PRACTICE EXAMINATION 1

SHORT ANSWER QUESTION PAPER 1

1. List the principal differential diagnoses of acute stridor in a 3-year-old child. Outline the management of life-threatening epiglottitis in a 3-year-old child.

2. A 40-year-old man is admitted with an acute head injury. List the indications for intubation, ventilation and referral to a neurosurgical unit.

3. Design a protocol for the management of massive intra-partum haemorrhage.

4. What information about benefits and side-effects do you give to a pregnant woman requesting epidural analgesic for relief of labour pain?

5. How would you investigate a patient with known cardiac ischaemia who is to undergo non-cardiac surgery?

6. Outline, with reasons, the management in the A&E Department of an elderly patient with a cherry-red face who has been found unconscious at home with a faulty gas heater.

7. Outline your management of an adult patient brought into the A&E Department in status asthmaticus.

8. What are the advantages and disadvantages of patient-controlled analgesia (PCA) for postoperative pain control?

9. Describe the principles behind the capnograph. What information can be obtained from this piece of monitoring equipment?

10. List the main complications that may occur during transurethral resection of the prostate, indicating how they might be dealt with.

11. Write a letter to a General Practitioner explaining how you would investigate and counsel a patient thought to have suffered from a hypersensitivity reaction to an anaesthetic drug.

12. Summarise the causes, effects and prevention of aspiration pneumonitis.

MULTIPLE CHOICE QUESTION PAPER 1

90 Questions: time allowed 3 hours.
Indicate your answers with a tick or cross in the spaces provided.

1.1 Trigeminal neuralgia

❑ A involves the 7th cranial nerve
❑ B is treated with radiofrequency ablation
❑ C is treated with glycerol injection
❑ D produces motor paralysis
❑ E is treated with carbamazepine

1.2 Concerning bilirubin metabolism

❑ A the diglucuronide is mostly formed in the liver
❑ B prior phenobarbitone treatment leads to enhanced conjugation
❑ C unconjugated bilirubin is damaging to the neonate
❑ D in haemolysis the bilirubin is mostly unconjugated
❑ E in extra-hepatic obstructive jaundice the bilirubin is mostly conjugated

1.3 Halothane

❑ A initially causes a reduction in respiratory rate
❑ B inhibits hypoxic pulmonary vasoconstriction
❑ C inhibits baroreceptors
❑ D is a bronchodilator
❑ E may cause a nodal bradycardia

1.4 When compared with fentanyl, alfentanil

❑ A has a greater volume of distribution
❑ B is more potent
❑ C causes more bradycardia
❑ D is more protein bound
❑ E has a longer elimination half-life

1.5 Platelet administration

- ❑ A needs filtration
- ❑ B needs cross-matching
- ❑ C causes significant increase in plasma histamine
- ❑ D contains citrate
- ❑ E platelets are viable after 2 weeks' storage

1.6 Pulmonary oedema is seen in

- ❑ A aortic stenosis
- ❑ B left atrial myxoma
- ❑ C massive pulmonary embolus
- ❑ D mitral stenosis
- ❑ E tricuspid stenosis

1.7 The following drugs are metabolised by cholinesterase:

- ❑ A mivacurium
- ❑ B esmolol
- ❑ C cocaine
- ❑ D bupivacaine
- ❑ E aspirin

1.8 The following drugs are effective transdermally:

- ❑ A morphine
- ❑ B fentanyl
- ❑ C atropine
- ❑ D hyoscine
- ❑ E glyceryl trinitrate (GTN)

1.9 The following are seen in chronic renal failure:

- ❑ A hypercalcaemia
- ❑ B hyponatraemia
- ❑ C hyperkalaemia
- ❑ D hypoproteinaemia
- ❑ E microcytic anaemia

1.10 A patient whose blood group is O Rh –ve has

- ❑ A anti-A agglutinin
- ❑ B anti-B agglutinin
- ❑ C anti-Rh agglutinin
- ❑ D anti-Kell antibodies
- ❑ E A and B agglutinogens

1.11 A young Afro-Caribbean boy needs open reduction and internal fixation of a fractured tibia. His Hb is 7.9 despite minimal blood loss. He should have

- ❑ A a sickledex test
- ❑ B transfusion of blood to a Hb of 10 g/dl pre-op
- ❑ C a tourniquet during the operation
- ❑ D hypotensive anaesthesia
- ❑ E cold intravenous fluids

1.12 In haemophilia A

- ❑ A there is a prolonged prothrombin time
- ❑ B there is polyarthropathy
- ❑ C gastrointestinal haemorrhage occurs
- ❑ D there is a deficiency of factor VIII
- ❑ E DDAVP may be given therapeutically

1.13 Hypotension during spinal anaesthesia may be caused by

- ❑ A bradycardia
- ❑ B autonomic blockade
- ❑ C hypovolaemia
- ❑ D aortocaval compression
- ❑ E anxiety

1.14 In effective basic life support during resuscitation

- ❑ A the inspired oxygen is 14%
- ❑ B the expired carbon dioxide is 2%
- ❑ C the pH of arterial blood should be > 7.4
- ❑ D the mixed venous oxygen saturation should be > 75%
- ❑ E the systolic blood pressure should be > 100 mmHg

1.15 In a 3.5 kg baby one would expect

- ❑ A a tidal volume of 60 ml
- ❑ B a blood volume of 20% of weight
- ❑ C anatomical dead space of 2 ml/kg
- ❑ D a Hb of 19 g/dl
- ❑ E a cardiac output of 1.5 l/min

1.16 Problems in Crohn's disease include

- ❑ A polyarthropathy
- ❑ B fistula in ano
- ❑ C entero-enteric fistulae
- ❑ D lymphoma
- ❑ E recurrence at operation site

1.17 Stellate ganglion block produces

- ❑ A mydriasis
- ❑ B postural hypotension
- ❑ C vasodilatation in the ipsilateral arm
- ❑ D reduced lacrimation
- ❑ E loss of the consensual light reflex

1.18 Postoperative hypertension is commonly due to

- ❑ A pain
- ❑ B hypocapnia
- ❑ C a full bladder
- ❑ D the residual effects of inhalation agents
- ❑ E phaeochromocytoma

1.19 You are called urgently to the labour ward by the obstetrician who has administered ergometrine. The uterus has contracted down and he cannot extract the second twin. The effects can be reversed by

- ❑ A halothane
- ❑ B thiopentone
- ❑ C salbutamol
- ❑ D ritodrine
- ❑ E suxamethonium

1.20 Suxamethonium is contraindicated in

- ❑ A dystrophia myotonica
- ❑ B acute intermittent porphyria
- ❑ C sickle cell disease
- ❑ D the neonate
- ❑ E congestive cardiac failure

1.21 Glutamine

❑ A is an essential amino acid
❑ B is a nutrient for enterocytes
❑ C is a nutrient for polymorphonuclear leucocytes
❑ D may be incorporated into total parental nutrition
❑ E allergy causes coeliac disease

1.22 Problems associated with laparoscopic surgery include

❑ A increased risk of regurgitation
❑ B gas embolism
❑ C pneumothorax
❑ D arrhythmias
❑ E shoulder tip pain

1.23 In total hip replacement

❑ A non-steroidal anti-inflammatory drugs may precipitate acute renal failure
❑ B regional techniques reduce long-term mortality
❑ C hypoxia intra-operatively may be due to embolism
❑ D hyperventilation is beneficial
❑ E methyl methacrylate is positively inotropic

1.24 The following nerves may be damaged in the lithotomy position:

❑ A common peroneal
❑ B femoral
❑ C obturator
❑ D saphenous
❑ E lateral cutaneous nerve of the thigh

1.25 Severe salicylate poisoning causes

❑ A thrombocytopenia
❑ B hypoprothrombinaemia
❑ C hypofibrinogenaemia
❑ D haemolysis
❑ E metabolic acidosis

1.26 The following occur in acute respiratory distress syndrome (ARDS):

❑ A decreased PaO_2
❑ B decreased $PaCO_2$
❑ C reduced lung compliance
❑ D reduced airway resistance
❑ E reduced diffusion capacity

1.27 The tachycardia produced by isoprenaline may be blocked by

❑ A atropine
❑ B nifedipine
❑ C phenobarbitone
❑ D propanolol
❑ E trimetaphan

1.28 Hepatitis B may be transmitted by

❑ A platelets
❑ B fibrinogen
❑ C albumin
❑ D plasma
❑ E packed red cells

1.29 The immediate treatment of anaphylaxis involves

- ❑ A adrenaline
- ❑ B ephedrine
- ❑ C chlorpheniramine
- ❑ D hydrocortisone
- ❑ E 0.9% saline

1.30 The femoral nerve

- ❑ A lies outside the femoral sheath
- ❑ B lies medial to the femoral artery
- ❑ C gives a cutaneous branch to the scrotum
- ❑ D is blocked in a '3:1' block
- ❑ E is a suitable block for fractured neck of femur

1.31 Hypotension following removal of a phaeochromocytoma is due to

- ❑ A acute adrenal failure
- ❑ B reduced intravascular volume
- ❑ C myocardial infarction
- ❑ D retroperitoneal haemorrhage
- ❑ E sepsis

1.32 Side-effects of amiodarone are

- ❑ A hypothyroidism
- ❑ B photosensitivity
- ❑ C corneal micro-deposits
- ❑ D peripheral neuropathy
- ❑ E pulmonary fibrosis

1.33 Characteristics of acute tubular necrosis are

❑ A malignant hypertension
❑ B a raised plasma urea but normal creatinine
❑ C concentrated urine
❑ D hyperkalaemia
❑ E a rapidly rising CVP

1.34 The following blood gases are seen with aspirin poisoning:

❑ A pH 6.9
❑ B $PaCO_2$ 3.2 kPa
❑ C PaO_2 10 kPa
❑ D actual bicarbonate of 10 mmol/l
❑ E readings consistent with a base excess of +5

1.35 Nitric oxide

❑ A is a bronchodilator
❑ B is synthesised from aspartamine
❑ C shows tachyphylaxis
❑ D is used therapeutically in a dose of 10–100 ppm
❑ E has an extremely high affinity for haemoglobin

1.36 A spinal block is contraindicated in

❑ A placenta praevia
❑ B pre-eclampsia
❑ C hypovolaemia
❑ D breech presentation
❑ E fetal distress

1.37 A tourniquet is applied to the leg for two hours. Signs of nerve damage include

- ❑ A extensor plantar
- ❑ B ankle clonus
- ❑ C reduced vibration sense at the ankle
- ❑ D reduced pin prick at the toe
- ❑ E reduced movement at the ankle after stimulation of the common peroneal nerve

1.38 Immediate problems following thyroidectomy include

- ❑ A hypocalcaemia
- ❑ B tracheal collapse
- ❑ C persistent laryngeal stridor
- ❑ D thyroid crisis
- ❑ E respiratory obstruction

1.39 A patient taking a MAOI suddenly develops a BP of 230/130 after being given ephedrine. Suitable treatment includes

- ❑ A labetalol
- ❑ B propranolol
- ❑ C phenobarbitone
- ❑ D diazoxide
- ❑ E guanethidine

1.40 Extrapyramidal side-effects are seen with

- ❑ A chlorpropramide
- ❑ B carbimazole
- ❑ C droperidol
- ❑ D metaclopramide
- ❑ E perphenazine

1.41 Propranolol

- ❑ A causes hyperglycaemia
- ❑ B causes reduced airway resistance
- ❑ C is contraindicated with verapamil
- ❑ D is the treatment of choice for post MI ventricular ectopics
- ❑ E causes selective blockade of beta-1 adrenergic receptors

1.42 Epidural anaesthesia is associated with the following:

- ❑ A an increased rate of instrumental delivery
- ❑ B headache
- ❑ C backache
- ❑ D urinary retention
- ❑ E deep vein thrombosis

1.43 Features of Down's syndrome include

- ❑ A atrial septal defect
- ❑ B trisomy 21
- ❑ C acute leukaemia
- ❑ D webbed neck
- ❑ E mental impairment

1.44 Medical complications of bronchial carcinoma include

- ❑ A peripheral neuropathy developing before diagnosis of the cancer
- ❑ B a common occurrence is lymphocytic meningitis
- ❑ C cerebellar degeneration without evidence of metastases
- ❑ D hypertrophic pulmonary osteoarthropathy
- ❑ E Horner's syndrome

1.45 Pulmonary artery occlusive pressure is a good guide to left ventricular end diastolic pressure in

- ❑ A cardiomyopathy
- ❑ B mitral stenosis
- ❑ C aortic incompetence
- ❑ D pulmonary stenosis
- ❑ E myocardial infarction

1.46 Prognostic indicators in ITU include

- ❑ A toe temperature
- ❑ B gastric blood flow
- ❑ C haematocrit
- ❑ D response to dobutamine
- ❑ E age of the patient

1.47 Endotoxin

- ❑ A is always found in septic patients
- ❑ B the test for its presence depends on crab's blood
- ❑ C a treatment for sepsis used antibody to the O antigen of endotoxin
- ❑ D may cause systemic hypotension
- ❑ E may cause pulmonary hypertension

1.48 Measurement of cardiac output using a pulmonary artery catheter is affected by

- ❑ A the temperature of the patient
- ❑ B the temperature of the injectate
- ❑ C position of the proximal port
- ❑ D constrictive pericarditis
- ❑ E the skill of the operator

1.49 In the ECG

- ❑ A the T wave represents ventricular depolarisation
- ❑ B K^+ is the major ion causing transmembrane potential
- ❑ C the QRS duration depends on the recording electrode
- ❑ D the V leads need only one recording electrode
- ❑ E a positive deflection occurs when depolarisation is going away from the recording electrode

1.50 The following suggest inadequate perfusion in posterior fossa surgery:

- ❑ A delta waves on EEG
- ❑ B arrhythmias
- ❑ C rise in BP
- ❑ D decrease in temperature
- ❑ E abnormal respiratory pattern

1.51 Propofol

- ❑ A produces green urine as a side-effect
- ❑ B causes less cardiac depression than thiopentone
- ❑ C is solubilised in egg phosphatide and glycerol emulsion
- ❑ D is 2,6 di-isopropyl phenol
- ❑ E is metabolised only in the liver

1.52 Wright's respirometer

- ❑ A is inaccurate at flows of < 1 l/min
- ❑ B is a turbine
- ❑ C is affected by viscosity of gas
- ❑ D is affected by humidity
- ❑ E can be used to measure peak flow

1.53 Nitrous oxide

- ❑ A is contraindicated in tympanoplasty
- ❑ B causes vitamin B12 deficiency
- ❑ C inhibits folate metabolism
- ❑ D is stored as a gas
- ❑ E is stored in blue cylinders

1.54 A fixed, low cardiac output occurs in

- ❑ A Paget's disease
- ❑ B Eisenmeger's syndrome
- ❑ C constrictive pericarditis
- ❑ D anaemia
- ❑ E aortic stenosis

1.55 A 'pink puffer', when compared with a 'blue bloater', will have

- ❑ A cor pulmonale
- ❑ B reduced sensitivity to respiratory drive from CO_2
- ❑ C a higher haematocrit
- ❑ D a lower PaO_2
- ❑ E a lower $PaCO_2$

1.56 Morbid obesity is associated with

- ❑ A reduced incidence of difficult intubation
- ❑ B an increased risk of regurgitation of acidic gastric contents
- ❑ C increased chest compliance
- ❑ D increased airways resistance
- ❑ E increased hypoxaemia during general anaesthesia

1.57 Peak flow

- ❑ A is not effort dependent
- ❑ B is measured by pneumotachograph
- ❑ C is measured by vitalograph
- ❑ D is reduced in acute asthma
- ❑ E has diurnal variation

1.58 In a patient with a flail chest, being ventilated, losing 1.5 l/min, treatment should include

- ❑ A reducing fresh gas flow by 1.5 l/min
- ❑ B adding 10 cm positive end expiratory pressure
- ❑ C reducing the peak inspiratory flow rate
- ❑ D increasing fresh gas flow by 1.5 l/min
- ❑ E inserting a chest drain

1.59 Concerning a pressure generator ventilator

- ❑ A it is a minute volume divider
- ❑ B inspiration – expiration can be time cycled
- ❑ C expiration – inspiration can be time cycled
- ❑ D reducing the flow rate enables better ventilation in bronchospasm
- ❑ E there is no risk of barotrauma

1.60 In paracetamol poisoning

- ❑ A N-acetylcysteine is a useful treatment
- ❑ B methionine is a useful treatment
- ❑ C jaundice is an early sign
- ❑ D prothrombin time is of prognostic value
- ❑ E liver transplant may be required

1.61 A supraclavicular brachial plexus block is more likely than an axillary block to produce

- ❑ A analgesia of shoulder
- ❑ B analgesia of fingers
- ❑ C a pneumothorax
- ❑ D intravascular injection
- ❑ E a Horner's syndrome

1.62 In the autonomic nervous system

- ❑ A acetylcholine is the neurotransmitter at all ganglia
- ❑ B noradrenaline is the neurotransmitter at postganglion sympathetic nerves
- ❑ C relaxation of the uterus is mediated by beta- 2 adrenoreceptors
- ❑ D beta adrenergic receptors are linked to adenylate cyclase
- ❑ E the action of noradrenaline is terminated mainly by metabolism

1.63 Regarding severe pre-eclampsia

- ❑ A magnesium sulphate is the anticonvulsant of choice
- ❑ B there may be a coagulopathy
- ❑ C normal vaginal delivery is usually possible
- ❑ D intravenous fluids are rarely necessary
- ❑ E general anaesthesia is the preferred type of anaesthetic if a caesarean section is required

1.64 The penicillins

- ❑ A are bacteriostatic
- ❑ B inhibit bacterial cell wall synthesis
- ❑ C are active only against Gram +ve organisms
- ❑ D rarely cause allergic reactions
- ❑ E are the treatment of choice for a UTI

1.65 Glycosuria occurs in

- ❑ A pregnancy
- ❑ B partial gastrectomy
- ❑ C head injury
- ❑ D phaeochromocytoma
- ❑ E acromegaly

1.66 Chronic renal failure is associated with

- ❑ A microcytic hypochromic anaemia
- ❑ B hypertension
- ❑ C bleeding disorder
- ❑ D a right shift of the oxygen-haemoglobin dissociation curve
- ❑ E secondary hyperparathyroidism

1.67 Suxamethonium is contraindicated

- ❑ A in acute renal failure
- ❑ B in Creutzfeld-Jakob disease
- ❑ C in dystrophia myotonica
- ❑ D in acute intermittent porphyria
- ❑ E the day after spinal cord injury

1.68 A thyroid storm may require treatment with

- ❑ A diazepam
- ❑ B propranolol
- ❑ C paracetamol
- ❑ D verapamil
- ❑ E chlorpromazine

1.69 The following anaesthetic agents are safe in a patient with acute porphyria:

❑ A methohexitone
❑ B suxamethonium
❑ C pancuronium
❑ D propofol
❑ E isoflurane

1.70 Thrombolytic therapy

❑ A is best accomplished with rTPA
❑ B is associated with malignant ventricular dysrrhythmias
❑ C should be combined with aspirin
❑ D can safely be performed within 24 hours of major surgery
❑ E cannot be repeated within three months with streptokinase

1.71 Sensory signs may occur with

❑ A carpal tunnel syndrome
❑ B tabes dorsalis
❑ C syringomyelia
❑ D motor neurone disease
❑ E multiple sclerosis

1.72 A fixed cardiac output state occurs with

❑ A constrictive pericarditis
❑ B mitral stenosis
❑ C patent ductus arteriosus
❑ D aortic stenosis
❑ E hypertrophic obstructive cardiomyopathy

1.73 Phantom limb pain

❑ A can be worsened by spinal anaesthesia
❑ B is worse if the limb is painful prior to amputation
❑ C incidence is reduced if epidural analgesia is established one week before amputation
❑ D may be treated with opioids
❑ E rarely responds to any form of therapy

1.74 A retrobulbar block will block the following:

❑ A short ciliary nerves
❑ B optic nerves
❑ C abducent nerve
❑ D facial nerve
❑ E oculomotor nerve

1.75 To suture a laceration on the palm of the hand the following should be blocked:

❑ A median nerve
❑ B ulnar nerve
❑ C musculocutaneous nerve
❑ D radial nerve
❑ E axillary nerve

1.76 The following are appropriate treatment regimens:

❑ A methionine for paraquat poisoning
❑ B assisted ventilation for salicylate poisoning
❑ C physostigmine for imipramine overdose
❑ D dicobalt edetate for cyanide poisoning
❑ E atropine for paracetamol poisoning

1.77 Concerning the Apgar score

- ❑ A it is valid in coloured babies
- ❑ B it is measured 1 minute after delivery of the head
- ❑ C it is a sensitive indicator of fetal distress
- ❑ D heart rate is as important as skin colour
- ❑ E muscle tone is not assessed

1.78 For amputation through the mid-thigh the following should be blocked:

- ❑ A femoral nerve
- ❑ B obturator nerve
- ❑ C lateral cutaneous nerve of the thigh
- ❑ D sciatic nerve
- ❑ E both sciatic and femoral nerve

1.79 A drug that blocks only dopamine receptors would be expected to

- ❑ A delay gastric emptying
- ❑ B reduce renal blood flow
- ❑ C reduce coronary blood flow
- ❑ D be useful in the treatment of Parkinson's disease
- ❑ E be an anti-emetic

1.80 A patient is likely to be successfully weaned from mechanical ventilation if

- ❑ A sedated
- ❑ B requiring an inspired oxygen concentration of 60%
- ❑ C the Pi max is > -30 cm H_2O
- ❑ D the chest X-ray shows pulmonary oedema
- ❑ E acidotic

1.81 In aortic regurgitation

- ❑ A angina only occurs when there is coexistent coronary atheroma
- ❑ B there is a systolic pressure gradient across the aortic valve
- ❑ C the murmur is best heard in the left lateral position
- ❑ D the stroke volume is three times normal
- ❑ E there is typically a diastolic thrill

1.82 Mannitol

- ❑ A is a sugar
- ❑ B is useful before biliary surgery
- ❑ C may cause circulatory overload
- ❑ D may cause neurological deterioration
- ❑ E is found in commercial preparations of dantrolene

1.83 Pulmonary fibrosis may occur with

- ❑ A bleomycin
- ❑ B paraquat
- ❑ C beryllium
- ❑ D cortisone hemisuccinate
- ❑ E amiodarone

1.84 Ulcerative colitis

- ❑ A is associated with cirrhosis
- ❑ B is associated with finger clubbing
- ❑ C is associated with cholangitis
- ❑ D is associated with carcinoma of the colon
- ❑ E rarely responds to steroids

1.85 Obstructive jaundice

❑ A causes high circulating levels of unconjugated bilirubin
❑ B leads to a high faecal fat level
❑ C is associated with an alkaline phosphatase level >100
❑ D leads to a high level of urobilinogen in the blood
❑ E may cause a coagulopathy

1.86 Negative nitrogen balance is found in

❑ A acute renal failure
❑ B post surgery
❑ C cortisone therapy
❑ D pregnancy
❑ E starvation

1.87 An asthmatic patient becomes wheezy towards the end of an anaesthetic; contributory factors may include

❑ A irritation of the trachea by an endotracheal tube
❑ B use of neostigmine
❑ C use of isoflurane
❑ D light anaesthesia
❑ E inclusion of morphine in the pre-medication

1.88 A raised reticulocyte count is found in

❑ A untreated megaloblastic anaemia
❑ B untreated iron deficiency
❑ C congenital spherocytosis
❑ D sickle cell trait
❑ E haemolysis

1.89 Pregnancy is associated with

- ❑ A reduced functional residual capacity
- ❑ B reduced vital capacity
- ❑ C increased airway resistance
- ❑ D increased alveolar ventilation
- ❑ E a hypercoaguable state

1.90 The following have been employed in the treatment of ARDS:

- ❑ A kinetotherapy
- ❑ B nitric oxide
- ❑ C nebulised prostacyclin
- ❑ D high frequency jet ventilation
- ❑ E IVOX

PRACTICE EXAM 1: THE CLINICAL VIVAS

Viva 1: The Clinical Viva takes place in the morning.

1. You are given a piece of clinical information and you have 10 minutes to study it.
2. You will spend 20 minutes with the first examiner, discussing the clinical care of the patient described and how you would anaesthetise for the case.
3. You will then spend 20 minutes with a second examiner discussing approximately three unrelated clinical scenarios.

Viva 2: The Clinical Science Viva takes place in the afternoon. Two examiners will question you for approximately 15 minutes each. Approximately four topics are covered.

A good way to prepare for the viva is to work with a partner. For this reason we have separated the sample questions in this book from the model answers to allow you to work through the viva session before looking at the answers.

Viva 1

Clinical Scenario

A 77-year-old lady is admitted for removal of cataract and insertion of an intraocular lens implant. She refuses local anaesthetic.

She suffered a myocardial infarct 9 years ago. She now only suffers infrequent angina for which she has a glyceryl trinitrate spray. Three years ago she had an operation because her right arm became pale, white and mottled.

Her current medications include warfarin, digoxin 0.125 mg mane and frumil one daily.

On examination the positive findings are a blowing pansystolic and early rumbling diastolic murmurs loudest at the apex. She has an irregularly irregular pulse and fine basal crepitations on auscultation of the lung fields. The apex beat is displaced in the 6th intercostal space in the anterior axillary line.

Her ECG and CXR are shown in Fig. 1 and Fig. 2 respectively.

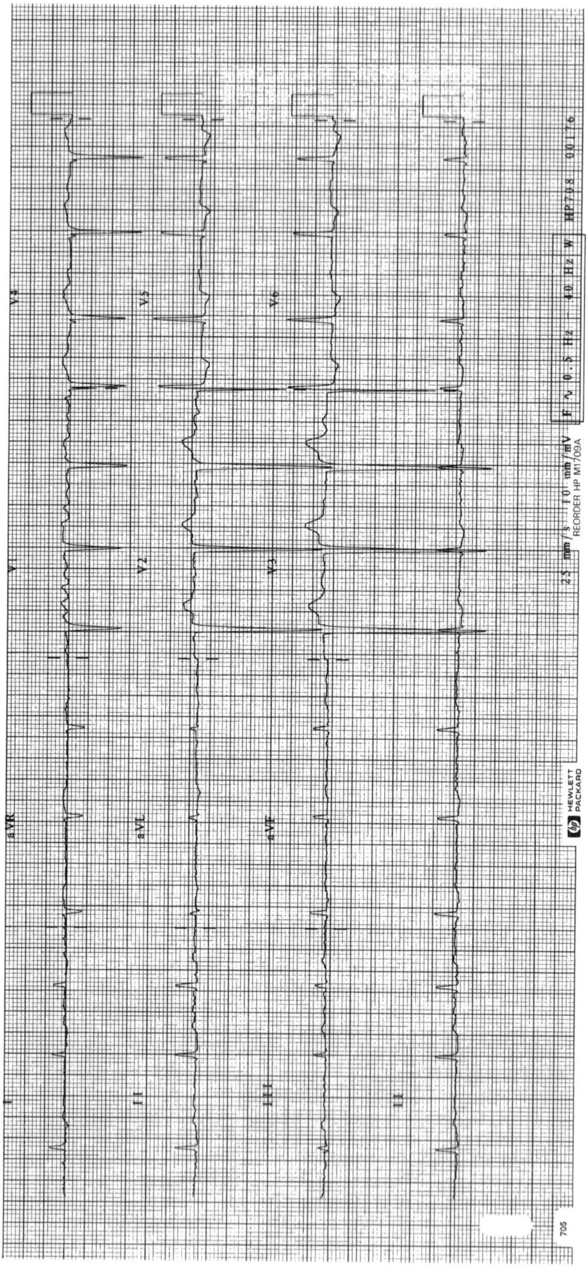

Fig. 1: ECG

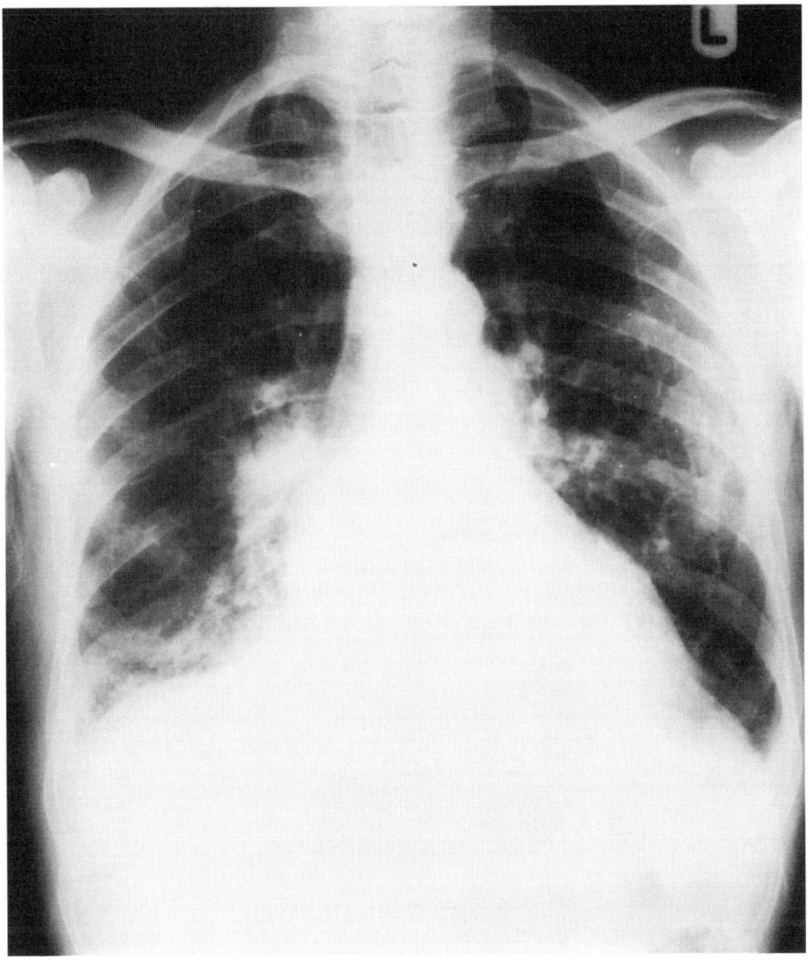

Fig. 2: Chest X-ray

Her biochemistry results are:

Na	140	Glucose	6.2		
K	5.5				
Urea	10				
Creatinine	140				
Hb	11.4	WCC	5.8	pt	256
INR	1.6				

Examiner 1

Summarise this lady's case.

Tell me about her ECG.

Describe the CXR.

Describe the cardiac outline, the lung fields and any obvious pathology.

How would you anaesthetise this lady?

Examiner 2

Tell me about premedication.

Tell me about the anaesthetic complications following thyroidectomy.

How would you anaesthetise a 25-year-old asthmatic who has a blood pressure of 170/100 and is due to have an inguinal hernia repair?

Viva 2

Examiner 1

Tell me about the anaemia of chronic renal failure.

Tell me about the causes of delayed gastric emptying.

Examiner 2

Tell me about the anatomy of the caudal canal.

Tell me about the problems of hypotensive anaesthesia.

SHORT ANSWER QUESTION PAPER 1 ANSWERS

1. ***List the principal differential diagnoses of acute stridor in a 3-year-old child. Outline the management of life-threatening epiglottitis in a 3-year-old child.***

Stridor is a high-pitched inspiratory noise characteristic of upper airway obstruction. The principal differential diagnoses are:

- Epiglottitis
- Croup
- Inhalation of foreign body
- Diphtheria
- Retropharyngeal abscess/haematoma
- Inhalation injury
- Trauma
- Angio neurotic oedema

Management of epiglottitis:

- Do not upset the child
- No IV access
- No neck X-ray
- Do not change the child's adopted sitting position and do not remove from parents
- Administer humidified oxygen, if feasible
- Call for senior help – anaesthetist/ENT surgeon/paediatrician
- Follow departmental guidelines for management:
  a) gas induction with oxygen and halothane in a safe environment – theatres/PICU
  b) minimal monitoring: ECG, oximeter, IV access
  c) secure airway with ETT when patient deeply anaesthetised – instruments available for tracheostomy
  d) capnograph to confirm satisfactory intubation
  e) blood cultures and other investigations to be sent – antibiotics administered – IV fluids given
  f) sedation for ventilation – pass a naso-gastric tube for feeding and oral sedative drugs – admit to Intensive Care Unit bed

2. ***A 40-year-old man is admitted with an acute head injury. List the indications for intubation, ventilation and referral to a neurosurgical unit.***

In a 40-year-old man who has sustained a head injury, the priorities are to avoid hypoxia, hypotension and hypercarbia to prevent secondary brain damage.

The indications for intubation and ventilation after head injury:

Immediately
- Coma (not obeying, not speaking, not eye opening), i.e. a Glasgow Coma Scale (GCS) ≤ 8
- Loss of protective laryngeal reflexes
- Ventilatory insufficiency (as judged by blood gases):
  a) hypoxaemia (PaO_2 < 9 kPa on air or < 13 kPa on oxygen)
  b) hypercarbia (PaO_2 > 6 kPa)
- Spontaneous hyperventilation causing $PaCO_2$ < 3.5 kPa
- Respiratory arrhythmias

Before transfer
- Significantly deteriorating conscious level, even if not in coma
- Bilaterally fractured mandible
- Copious bleeding into mouth (e.g. from skull base fracture)
- Seizures

An intubated patient must be ventilated. Aim for PaO_2 > 15 kPa, PaO_2 4–4.5 kPa.

The criteria for referring head-injured patients to a neurosurgical unit:

Immediately (after initial assessment and resuscitation)
- Fractured skull, with any of the following:
  a) any alteration of conscious level (GCS < 15)
  b) focal neurological signs
  c) fits
  d) any other neurological symptoms/signs
- Coma persisting after resuscitation – even without a skull fracture
- Deterioration of conscious level – even without a skull fracture
- Focal pupil or limb signs – even without a skull fracture

Urgently (not necessarily immediately)

- Confusion persisting > 6 hours (even without a skull fracture)
- Compound depressed skull fracture (or other penetrating injury)
- Suspected leak of CSF from nose or ear
- Persistent or worsening headache or vomiting (especially in a child)

Ref: BMJ 1993: 307; 547–552.

3. ***Design a protocol for the management of massive intra-partum haemorrhage.***

The definition of massive intra-partum haemorrhage is more than 1 ml/kg/minute blood loss. The main aim is to initiate resuscitation, to enrol senior help and transfer the patient to theatre as soon as possible.

- If the patient is undelivered, put in left lateral position. Administer oxygen
- Ask for senior anaesthetist/obstetrician/midwife
- Establish IV access with 2 x 14 G cannulae
- Send bloods at the same time for cross-matching, FBC, clotting
- Inform the blood bank
- Administer colloid with a pressurised giving set
- With every 6 units of blood, give platelets and FFP via a fluid warmer
- Get control of bleeding by going to theatre
- Post-partum haemorrhage may be due to retention of the products of conception. Therefore, consider syntocinon or ergometrine
- Monitor basic parameters, coagulation status, if undelivered, the fetal heart rate, and monitor central venous pressure
- Give O-neg blood if cross-matched blood not easily available
- Consider Intensive Care Unit bed for the patient.

4. *What information about benefits and side-effects do you give to a pregnant woman requesting epidural analgesia for relief of labour pain?*

The benefits of epidural analgesia:
- Analgesia superior to either entonox, intramuscular pethidine or TENS
- Easily performed, generally effective with minimal serious side-effects to either mother or fetus
- If necessary can be used for instrumental delivery (forceps, ventouse) or for caesarean section

The commonest side-effects include:
- Hypotension, avoided by pre-loading with IV fluid
- Pruritis if opiates are used. Rarely troublesome. Many respond to a small dose of naloxone (40 μg) or propofol (10–20 mg)
- Shivering

These are due to autonomic blockade.
- Dural puncture – occurs in about 1:200 patients. It causes severe headache and may require epidural blood patch.

Less common problems which one may not wish to burden the mother with include:
- Urinary retention
- High epidural block
- Inadvertent intravascular injection of local anaesthetic

It is worth informing the mother that there is an increased chance of her requiring an instrumental delivery with an epidural. The question of whether there is an increased rate of caesarean section after an epidural is sited remains debatable.

Ref: Fetal & Maternal Med Review 1996: 8; 29–55.

5. ***How would you investigate a patient with known cardiac ischaemia who is to undergo non-cardiac surgery?***

Preoperative investigation of ischaemic heart disease

Standard investigations:

- FBC: Anaemia, which further compromises coronary oxygen supply, should be excluded
- CXR: A routine CXR should be performed to exclude cardiac failure
- 12 lead ECG: This may be normal or show ST segment or T wave abnormalities indicating ischaemia. Evidence of previous myocardial infarct, rhythm disturbance or conduction abnormality may be present

Specialised investigations:

- Exercise stress test: the ECG is continuously monitored while the patient undergoes graded exercise on a treadmill. Although a negative stress test is encouraging it does not exclude coronary artery disease.
- Radionuclear imaging:
  a) *Thallium scanning*: Thallium is taken up after intravenous injection by viable myocardium. A fixed defect or 'cold spot' indicates infarcted myocardium whereas reversible defects represent ischaemia.
  b) *Dipyridamole thallium scanning (DTI)*: Dipyridamole is used to induce coronary vasodilation pharmacologically after which thallium scanning is performed.
  c) *MUGA scan*: the isotope technetium-99 is used. This technique assesses left ventricular ejection fraction, stroke volume and regional wall motion abnormalities.
- Echocardiography: provides information about the heart valves, stroke volume and ejection fraction. It can show areas of dyskinesis and regional wall motion abnormalities due to ischaemic or infarcted myocardium.
- Cardiac catheterization: although this is an invasive procedure, it remains the gold standard for the demonstration of coronary artery disease.

Ref: BJA 1994: 74; 104–116.

6. ***Outline, with reasons, the management in the A&E Department of an elderly patient with a cherry-red face who has been found unconscious at home with a faulty gas heater.***

Initial management of this patient should involve basic resuscitation – checking the airway (applying high concentration of oxygen), breathing and circulation. A history should be obtained and the patient examined for associated injuries. The main problem appears to be that of carbon monoxide (CO) poisoning and this should be determined by sending blood not only for FBC, U&E and arterial blood gases but also for CO estimation on a laboratory co-oximeter. Other investigations should include a chest X-ray and ECG.

Carbon monoxide poisoning may present with symptoms of headache and nausea at levels of 15–20% progressing to coma at levels > 40%. CO binds haemoglobin 250 times more avidly than oxygen hence reducing oxygen carriage by the blood. Additionally, it causes a leftwards shift of the oxygen dissociation curve and poisons the mitochondrial enzymes, causing a metabolic acidosis.

Measurement is only by a co-oximeter as the IR absorption of CO causes pulse oximeters to read towards 96% saturation.

Treatment involves protection of the airway if the patient is unconscious (GCS < 8) and ventilation with 100% oxygen. This reduces the half-life of CO from 4 hours to 45 minutes. In the unconscious patient, hyperbaric oxygen is also useful but centres with the facility for IPPV in the hyperbaric chamber are rare. Monitoring should include ECG, blood pressure and $ETCO_2$. The cardiovascular system may require support, the metabolic acidosis may require management with bicarbonate if severe but this is controversial. Finally, other injuries should be sought and treated appropriately.

7. ***Outline your management of an adult patient brought into the A&E Department in status asthmaticus.***

Acute severe asthma (or status asthmaticus) is a medical emergency.

Clinical signs indicating severe attack:
- Inability to speak
- Respiratory rate > 25/min
- Tachycardia > 110/min
- Pulsus paradoxus > 10 mmHg
- PaO_2 < 8 kPa
- $PaCO_2$ > 6.5 kPa

Particularly ominous signs:
- Silent chest on auscultation
- Cyanosis
- Bradycardia, hypotension (< 90 mmHg systolic)
- Confusion
- Exhaustion, respiratory rate > 50 or < 10

Consider ventilation if:
- PaO_2 < 8 kPa (despite $FiO_2 \geq 0.6$)
- $PaCO_2$ > 6 kPa
- pH < 7.3

Prior to transfer to Intensive Care Unit:
- Give highest possible inspired oxygen concentration by mask.
- Insert intravenous cannula; 0.5–1 litre intravenous fluids as often dehydrated. Intubate (rapid sequence induction) and ventilate.
- Pharmacological treatment:
  a) nebulised salbutamol every 2–4 hours, 5 mg in 5 ml saline in 100% oxygen. Switch to intravenous salbutamol if no response.
  b) nebulised ipratropium bromide every 6 hours, 0.5 mg in 5 ml saline in 100% oxygen.
  c) intravenous aminophylline
     i) Loading dose (except in patients on regular oral theophyllines) 5 mg/kg over 15–30 minutes. Signs of toxicity are hypotension, arrhythmias and convulsions.
     ii) Maintenance dose 0.5–0.9 mg/kg/hr. Narrow therapeutic index. Monitor levels regularly (therapeutic range 10–20 mg/l).
  d) intravenous hydrocortisone 200 mg bolus, repeat every 6 hours.
  e) antibiotics if signs of infection (purulent sputum, fever, leucocytosis).

- Further investigations: CXR, ECG, repeat arterial blood gases, FBC including WBC, serum potassium.
- Ventilation:
  i) aim is to oxygenate adequately
  ii) avoid barotrauma
  iii) permissive hypercapnia
  iv) use prolonged expiratory phase
  v) physiotherapy to clear secretions

Assess response to therapy:
- Clinically
- Blood gases: PaO_2 and $PaCO_2$
- Airway pressures

8. *What are the advantages and disadvantages of patient controlled analgesia (PCA) for postoperative pain control?*

PCA is a form of postoperative pain control which has been in use in many hospitals over the last 5–8 years. It involves the intravenous admission of boluses delivered by a syringe pump triggered by the patient. The pump is set up by the anaesthetist, the amount of analgesia timed between boluses (lock-out). Maximum dose in 4 hours and the possibility of a background infusion are all set before use. The advantages of this method of postoperative analgesia are numerous. Possibly the most important is the fact that the patient controls his/her own pain relief. Studies have shown that patient satisfaction has increased because of this. A major advantage is that the patient does not have to wait for a nurse to get the drug, check with another nurse and then administer it. The other benefits are that the drug is delivered intravenously as opposed to intramuscularly, and small and regular boluses are given as opposed to large infrequent doses leading to a more constant plasma level and implicit safety. Safety is important. The patient controls his own level of analgesia and if he is sleepy he will not press the button; therefore, if used correctly, overdoses are extremely unlikely. Finally, other drugs can be included in the PCA such as anti-emetics to control nausea.

The disadvantages are that there is, of course, a potential for malfunction of the pump and, therefore, the delivery of a potentially fatal dose of opiate to the patient. The syringe pump should be attached to the patient by a specialised giving set which has an anti-syphon valve and a one-way valve so that if an intravenous infusion is connected to the patient there can be no risk of the narcotic backing up into the intravenous set.

On the practical side, the button may be difficult to press if the patient has had hand or arm surgery and does not have the strength to push the button; this is particularly relevant with the elderly. The pumps are not suitable for those who cannot understand how to use them and, therefore, in any patients who are confused or children less than 5–6 years of age. Side-effects of the narcotic are nausea, itching, ileus and hallucinations. Patients are not 'pain-free' as with a regional technique. Some patients are unable to understand the need or are reluctant to operate the button. Mobility is restricted because of the pump, drip pole, etc.

In general, this form of analgesia is a major advance in postoperative pain control as long as it is set up correctly and is used correctly by the patient and not by their relatives.

9. Describe the principles behind the capnograph. What information can be obtained from this piece of monitoring equipment?

The capnograph is used to monitor end-tidal carbon dioxide ($ETCO_2$). It employs the Luft principle which states that any molecule with two or more different atoms will absorb infra-red radiation. It is thus an infra-red spectrophotometer.

The following information can be obtained:

- Respiratory rate
- Adequacy of ventilation
- The $ETCO_2$ approximates to $PaCO_2$ which provides an assessment of adequacy of ventilation. Hypoventilation causes a raised $ETCO_2$, hyperventilation a reduced $ETCO_2$
- Indirect assessment of cardiac output
  Presence of expired CO_2 ($ETCO_2$) depends on adequate lung perfusion which in turn depends on the cardiac output. In low cardiac output states the $ETCO_2$ will be low. In cardiac arrest there is no capnograph trace.
- Disconnection alarm
  In event of disconnection of breathing system/ventilator the capnograph trace will disappear.
- Confirmation of correct placement of ET tube
  The only totally reliable way of confirming tracheal placement of an ET tube is by a consistent, normal capnograph waveform.
- Detection of malignant hyperpyrexia
  In MH the earliest signs are tachycardia, desaturation and an elevated and rising $ETCO_2$ (as well as temperature).
- Detection of pulmonary embolus
- Pulmonary embolus (air, fat, cement, thrombosis) produces a sudden decline in $ETCO_2$ (in conjunction with desaturation and hypotension)
- Indirect assessment of neuromuscular block
  In the absence of a peripheral nerve stimulator, the capnograph trace may indicate when the neuromuscular block wears off and the patient tries to breathe.
- Detection of re-breathing
  In, for example, inadequate fresh gas flow or exhausted soda lime in a circle system.
- Detection of bronchospasm
  The capnograph is altered in patients with chronic airflow limitation and also if bronchospasm develops intra-operatively.

10. List the main complications that may occur during transurethral resection of the prostate, indicating how they might be dealt with.

Complications that occur during transurethral resection of the prostate (TURP) may be general (i.e. those of an elderly population undergoing anaesthesia and surgery) or specific to that operation.

General

- *Cardiovascular*. These elderly patients are at an increased risk of CVS morbidity and mortality. Ischaemia, myocardial infarction, hypotension and arrhythmias may all be encountered.
- *Respiratory*. Chronic pulmonary disease is also relatively common and this may be exacerbated by lithotomy position. Regional anaesthesia may improve outcome. Pulmonary aspiration is always a potential risk.
- *Other*. There may be deterioration in renal function particularly on a background of chronic renal impairment. Neurological problems may arise ranging from confusion to cerebral infarction.

Specific

- *TUR syndrome*. This is a clinical syndrome of confusion, cardiovascular instability (hypertension, arrhythmias, pulmonary oedema) and subsequent unconsciousness and seizure activity. Underlying pathophysiology: absorption of glycine solution used to irrigate the operative field (related to height of the bags, operator skill and duration of the operation). The patient becomes overloaded with water causing the haemodynamic instability and hyponatraemia causing some of the CVS disturbances (glycine toxicity also contributes). Treatment is supportive. Fluid replacement with N saline and frusemide used to reduce the intravascular water load. Early detection is important and hence regional anaesthesia is often used.
- *Bladder rupture*. Presents as abdominal pain. Shock and features of excessive water absorption may follow. Treatment is surgical repair and supportive.
- *Bleeding*. This may be excessive both because of excessive gland vascularity and release of fibrinolytic substances such as urokinase. Treatment is supportive. Bleeding is reduced by regional anaesthesia. Occasionally anti-fibrinolytic therapy with tranexamic acid or aprotinin may be required in conjunction with blood products such as fresh frozen plasma and platelets.
- *Sepsis*. Bacteraemia may result from the instrumentation of a chronically catheterised urinary tract. Treatment is supportive in conjunction with suitable (Gram-negative) antibiotics.
- *Diathermy burns*.

11. Write a letter to a General Practitioner explaining how you would investigate and counsel a patient thought to have suffered from a hypersensitivity reaction to an anaesthetic drug.

Dear Dr

Re:

Thank you for your letter of .... regarding this patient who may have had a hypersensitivity reaction to an anaesthetic drug.

I am not sure whether the appropriate serum samples were taken at the time of reaction and at intervals afterwards. I will arrange to see the patient and try to gain as accurate a history of the event as possible.

As far as testing the patient now, I shall arrange for his/her admission for skin testing for the suspected drugs. This involves making a small subcutaneous injection of a dilute (starting in 1:100 dilution) sample of the relevant drugs. This is still the most reliable method although it does carry a small risk of further reaction and full resuscitative equipment is always present. In discussion with the Immunologists we may also consider radio-allergosorbent (RAST) testing, or latex agglutination testing. The hope is that we can identify the drug responsible for the reaction and subsequently inform yourself, make the notes and of course, explain all of this to the patient him/herself, encouraging him/her to wear an appropriate 'medic alert' type bracelet and carry a card documenting the drug(s) to be avoided. If this is so your patient can be reassured that anaesthesia undertaken in the absence of the drug(s) responsible should be quite safe.

It is often not possible to identify the specific drug responsible accurately as several drugs are given at induction of anaesthesia. If this is the case, we can still avoid the most likely drugs and use only those drugs known to carry a very low incidence of adverse reaction. Some would also recommend H_1- and H_2-antagonist with a corticosteroid with the pre-med.

Yours

12. Summarise the causes, effects and prevention of aspiration pneumonitis.

Aspiration pneumonitis is due to pulmonary damage from aspiration of acidic gastric contents.

Factors predisposing to regurgitation:
- *Full stomach*
- *Delayed gastric emptying.* Anxiety, trauma, obesity, pain, diabetes, alcohol, opioids and anticholinergic drugs
- *Reduced lower oesophageal pressure.* Hiatus hernia, pregnancy, atropine, opioids

The effects of aspiration:
- Mild cases: reduced oxygen saturation, wheezing or coughing
- Severe cases: respiratory failure and ARDS may develop requiring artificial ventilation.

Prevention:

Elective surgery
- No solids for 6 hours, no fluids for 4 hours prior to anaesthesia
- Consider awake intubation or regional technique.

Emergency surgery – the following may be considered:
- Nasogastric tube to drain stomach contents
- H_2 receptor antagonists or omeprazole to reduce the acidity of gastric contents
- Metaclopramide or cisapride to promote gastric emptying Metaclopramide also increases lower oesophageal sphincter tone.
- Sodium citrate or other non-particulate antacid to reduce the pH of stomach contents
- Preoxygenation and rapid sequence induction – this secures the airway rapidly
- Cricoid pressure – this manoeuvre compresses the oesophagus between cricoid cartilage and vertebrae and prevents onward passage of any regurgitated material
- Extubate the patient only when he is fully awake with protective laryngeal reflexes present
- Awake intubation or regional technique if feasible.

Ref: Hospital Update: May 1994. Aspiration and its prevention.

MCQ PAPER 1 ANSWERS

1.1 Trigeminal neuralgia **Answers: B C E**

Trigeminal neuralgia is an agonising pain in the distribution of the trigeminal (fifth) cranial nerve, usually triggered from a place on the lips or the side of the nose. It is purely sensory, usually unilateral and does not affect the corneal reflex. It occurs mainly in the elderly; in a patient under fifty years old it may be symptomatic of multiple sclerosis. It may be relieved by carbamazepine or phenytoin. If medical therapy fails the patient may need phenol or glycerol injection into, section or radiofrequency ablation of the trigeminal nerve. The pain may be so severe that the patient commits suicide.

1.2 Bilirubin metabolism **Answers: A B C D E**

Bilirubin is formed in the liver from the breakdown of redundant red blood cells. Unconjugated bilirubin is initially formed. The neonate may be damaged if unconjugated bilirubin crosses the immature blood–brain barrier, causing kernicterus (damage to the basal ganglia). In haemolysis there is an increase in unconjugated bilirubin and no bile in the urine. Bilirubin is conjugated in the hepatocytes and excreted in the bile mainly as the diglucuronide. Conjugation is enhanced by phenobarbitone by induction of the hepatic cytochrome P450 enzyme system. Extra-hepatic jaundice is characterised by pale stools and dark urine. The bilirubin is conjugated.

1.3 Halothane **Answers: B C D E**

Halothane is a halogenated hydrocarbon. Its chemical formula is 2-bromo, 2-chloro, 1, 1, 1,-trifluoroethane. It has a MAC of 0.76, a blood gas solubility coefficient of 2.4, a boiling point of 50 degrees Celsius, and a saturated vapour pressure of 32 kPa. It is unstable in light and therefore stored in dark bottles. It contains 0.01% thymol as a preservative. It is a bronchodilator and after sevoflurane is the least irritant to the respiratory tract of all the volatile agents. It inhibits hypoxic vasoconstriction, as do all the volatile agents.

It is a potent depressant of myocardial contractility. It may cause a nodal bradycardia, and in addition sensitises the myocardium to the action of catecholamines, arrhythmias are common. Halothane causes hypotension and inhibits the baroreceptor reflex, preventing a compensatory tachycardia. Halothane is 20% metabolised by the liver.

In up to 25% of patients exposed to halothane, there may be a mild, subclinical hepatitis, with jaundice and elevated liver enzymes. Rarely, a fulminating hepatic necrosis may occur which has a high mortality.

1.4 Pharmacokinetics of alfentanil and fentanyl **Answer: D**

Alfentanil has a smaller volume of distribution (Vd) and a lower pKa than fentanyl. It therefore has a faster onset, and a shorter duration of action. Alfentanil is less potent as it is less lipid soluble. Alfentanil is 92% protein bound, while fentanyl is 84% protein bound.

1.5 Platelet administration **Answers: A D**

Platelets may be transfused to patients with acute thrombocytopenia, for instance in the context of postoperative bleeding. Platelets should be administered using a special filter. They do not require cross-matching, but must be group compatible. Platelets contain citrate as an anti-coagulant. Although platelets contain histamine, platelet administration does not result in any significant increase in plasma histamine. Platelets have a short shelf life, and need to be administered within a few days of collection.

1.6 Pulmonary oedema **Answers: B D**

Pulmonary oedema occurs when the left atrial pressure is elevated. This may occur in such diverse conditions as mitral stenosis and left atrial myxoma.

1.7 Plasma cholinesterases **Answers: A B C E**

Several anaesthetic agents are metabolised by plasma cholinesterases. Suxamethonium is the best known example, but all the ester local anaesthetics, including cocaine, are also metabolised this way. Mivacurium, a non-depolarising muscle relaxant and esmolol, a short-acting beta blocker, undergo metabolism by cholinesterases. So does aspirin!

Ref: Anaesthesia 1997: 52; 244–260.

1.8 Transdermal drugs **Answers: B D E**

Many drugs can be administered transdermally. Glyceryl trinitrate is often administered as small patches. Hyoscine patches are used as a treatment for motion sickness. Transdermal fentanyl patches are available for pain control in cancer patients.

1.9 Chronic renal failure **Answers: A B C D E**

The patient with chronic renal failure is almost invariably anaemic. The anaemia is usually normocytic. The anaemia would only be hypochromic and microcytic if there was associated iron deficiency, due, for example, to chronic occult blood loss. The anaemia of chronic renal failure is due

to lack of erythropoietin production by the kidneys. There is often a bleeding tendency due to platelet dysfunction, although the platelet count is often normal. Hypogastrinaemia and peptic ulceration occur.
There is usually hypocalcaemia with associated hyperphosphataemia. The kidney is responsible for the conversion of 25-hydroxy cholecalciferol (made in the liver) to the active metabolite 1,25-dihydroxycholecalciferol (1,25(OH)2D3). The absorption of calcium from the gut requires 1,25(OH)2D3; in its absence hypocalcaemia occurs. Hypocalcaemia leads to secondary hyperparathyroidism, renal osteodystrophy and hypercalcaemia. The serum albumin is reduced if there is nephrotic syndrome. The serum sodium is normal up to the very terminal stage of chronic renal failure.

1.10 The rhesus system **Answers: A B**

The rhesus system describes the presence of (rhesus positive) or absence of (rhesus negative) the rhesus antigen on the surface of the red blood cells. The ABO system is the other major red cell antigen system used in transfusion medicine. A patient who is blood group O rhesus-negative has neither A, B or rhesus antigens on the surface of their blood cells. They are thus the universal donor, as the lack of red antigens precludes any immunological response by a recipient. Because O rhesus-negative patients have no red cell antigens they therefore recognise A, B and rhesus as foreign and therefore have anti-A and anti-B antibodies (agglutinins) in their serum. Rhesus antibodies, however, only result from previous transfusion or pregnancy.
The Kell antigen is part of a lesser antigen system: the Kell, Kidd and Duffy system. There is no reason why an O rhesus-negative patient should have anti-Kell antibodies.

1.11 Sickle cell disease **Answer: A**

A low haemoglobin in the absence of significant blood loss in an Afro-Caribbean male points to a possible diagnosis of sickle cell disease. The diagnosis is easily confirmed by a sickledex test, which will, if positive, confirm the presence of sickle haemoglobin (Hb S). To quantify the amount of Hb S, haemoglobin electrophoresis is necessary.
The gene coding for abnormal sickle haemoglobin is inherited in simple Mendelian fashion. Heterozygotes for the gene are said to have sickle cell trait, while the homozygous state is termed sickle cell disease. Sickle cell trait is a benign condition, the Hb is normal and the amount of Hb S present is 25–45%. Sickle cell disease is a severe haemolytic anaemia. The amount of Hb S is 85–95%; there is no normal Hb A present. There is marked anaemia with a Hb of 6–9 g/dl. The peripheral blood film is

grossly abnormal with sickle cells and target cells present. Patients with sickle cell disease suffer repeated painful crises, due to the occlusion of the microvasculature in the bones by the sickle cells.

At the molecular level sickle haemoglobin is due to a single base change in the DNA coding for the amino acid in position 6 in the beta chain of Hb. The result is that sickle haemoglobin forms insoluble crystals in hypoxic conditions. The red blood cells become sickle shaped and tend to occlude the microvasculature especially in the bones, leading to the painful crises.

In anaesthetic terms, the patient should be kept well hydrated. Hypothermia, hypoxia, hypotension, acidosis and venous stasis should be avoided as these predispose to red cell sickling. Tourniquets and even blood pressure cuffs, can cause sickling in the limb on which they are applied.

For major surgery an exchange transfusion may be carried out preoperatively. The aim is to reduce the level of Hb S to less than 30% to reduce the chance of sickling in the perioperative period. Transfusion to a preoperative Hb of 10 g/dl in a patient with a Hb of 7.9 g/dl is unnecessary and potentially hazardous. Because the anaemia is chronic, there is a compensatory shift of the oxygen/haemoglobin dissociation curve to enable adequate tissue oxygen extraction. Transfused blood is deficient in 2,3 DPG and so actually impairs tissue oxygenation. Blood transfusion will also increase blood viscosity and make sickling more likely.

Ref: BJA 1998: 80; 820–828.

1.12 Haemophilia **Answers: B C D E**

Haemophilia is an X-linked recessive haemorrhagic disorder. It is due to deficiency of clotting factor number 8 (factor VIII). As factor VIII is part of the intrinsic clotting cascade the partial thromboplastin time (APTT) is prolonged, while the prothrombin time (PT) is normal. The platelet count is normal.

Clinically, patients often suffer recurrent painful haemarthroses and muscle haematomas. Prolonged bleeding may occur after circumcision or dental extractions. Haematuria and gastrointestinal haemorrhage may occur. The severity of clinical symptoms depends on the level of factor VIII activity.

Haemophiliacs are treated with regular injections of factor VIII. This used to be supplied from heat-treated pooled serum donations, but factor

VIII is now made from recombinant DNA technology which prevents the risk of transmission of HIV or hepatitis C. Factor VIII levels can also effectively be raised by the administration of desmopressin (DDAVP) or cryoprecipitate.

1.13 Spinal anaesthesia **Answers: A B C D**

Spinal anaesthesia results in loss of the vasoconstrictor tone in the circulation in the lower limbs, due to autonomic blockade. This may lead to hypotension, which can be counteracted by the administration of intravenous fluid (preloading), or by a vasoconstrictor such as ephedrine or methoxamine. If the spinal block is high enough to block the cardiac accelerator fibres (T1–T4) bradycardia occurs leading to hypotension which may be corrected by atropine or glycopyrrolate. In obstetric anaesthesia it is important to avoid aortocaval compression, which, in combination with a spinal, may lead to profound hypotension.

Ref: BJA 1993: 70; 672–680.

1.14 Effective cardiopulmonary resuscitation **Answer: A**

In effective mouth-to-mouth resuscitation, the percentage inspired oxygen is about 14%. The expired CO_2 (i.e. the patient's) will be much greater than 2% because they are likely to have been apnoeic for some time.

The patient will have both a respiratory and metabolic acidosis: due to apnoea and anaerobic tissue metabolism, respectively. The pH of the blood will be less than 7.4, which is the normal plasma pH. The mixed venous oxygen saturation (SvO_2) in a normal individual is about 75%. In a patient receiving effective mouth-to-mouth resuscitation the SvO_2 would be unlikely to be greater than 75%. It is extremely unlikely that the systolic blood pressure will be anything approaching 100 mmHg.

1.15 A 3.5 kg baby **Answers: C D E**

In a neonate, the tidal volume is 5–7 mg/kg. Dead space is about 2–3 ml/kg. Blood volume is 80–100 ml/kg (i.e. about 10% of body weight). The haemoglobin concentration at birth is about 18 g/dl. This rises by about 1.2 g/dl in the first week. It then declines to around 10 g/dl at 3 months. By the first year it is about 12 g/dl and thereafter increases until adolescence.

1.16 Crohn's disease **Answers: A B C D E**

Crohn's disease is a granulomatous condition of unknown aetiology. It can affect any part of the gastrointestinal tract from mouth to anus, but most commonly affects the terminal ileum. It commonly presents with abdominal pain and diarrhoea. A low grade fever, weight loss, anaemia, polyarthropathy, uveitis, skin rashes (erythema nodosum and pyoderma gangrenosum) can all occur. Lymphoma may develop in affected bowel. Fistula in ano and entero - enteric fistulae are not uncommon. Medical treatment includes the use of corticosteroids, azathioprine and sulphasalazine. Surgery is often necessary, but unfortunately recurrence at the site of operation is not unusual.

1.17 Stellate ganglion block **Answer: C**

A stellate ganglion block produces:

a) a Horner's syndrome, ptosis, enophthalmos, miosis
b) temperature increase in the ipsilateral arm and hand due to vasodilatation
c) flushing of the conjunctiva and skin
d) nasal stuffiness.

There is not sufficient sympathetic blockade to produce postural hypotension. The light reflex involves the optic nerve and the parasympathetic fibres of the oculomotor nerve and so is unaffected by a stellate ganglion block.

1.18 Postoperative hypertension **Answers: A C**

There are numerous possible causes of postoperative hypertension. The common causes include:

a) pain, inadequate analgesia
b) pre-existing hypertension, inadequately treated or as yet undiagnosed
c) hypothermia, hypoxia or hypercarbia
d) a full bladder.

Although phaeochromocytoma is a cause of postoperative hypertension it is extremely uncommon.

1.19 Action of drugs on the uterus **Answers: A C D**

The uterus consists of smooth muscle and therefore receives its motor innervation from the autonomic nervous system. There is no striated muscle and so neither suxamethonium nor any of the non-depolarising neuromuscular blocking drugs will have any effect on the uterus. The sympathetic outflow to the uterus comes from L2, L3 and L4. The uterus is also affected by the hormone oxytocin from the posterior pituitary. Oxytocin causes contraction of the uterus. The synthetic equivalent is

generally used in obstetric anaesthetic practice. Syntocinon also causes tachycardia and hypotension. Prostaglandins will cause contraction of the uterus.
The action of sympathetic nerves on the uterus is via beta-2 receptors. Salbutamol and ritodrine both stimulate beta-2 receptors causing uterine relaxation. These agents can therefore be used to antagonise the effects of ergometrine. Halothane, like all the volatile agents causes uterine relaxation.

1.20 Contraindications to suxamethonium **Answer: A**

The unwanted effects of suxamethonium include:
a) myalgia postoperatively
b) hyperkalaemia
c) malignant hyperthermia
d) anaphylaxis
e) suxamethonium apnoea.

In terms of contraindications, a patient known to have allergy to suxamethonium, and patients in whom hyperkalaemia would be especially dangerous should not receive the drug. There are a number of myopathic conditions in which suxamethonium is contraindicated. Dystrophia myotonica is one such condition, as is myotonia congenita. There is increased sensitivity to the drug in the Eaton-Lambert syndrome, and it should be avoided.

Suxamethonium does not precipitate porphyria, nor is it contraindicated in sickle cell disease, the neonate or in congestive cardiac failure.

1.21 Glutamine **Answers: B D**

Glutamine is a non-essential amino acid, although in times of physiological stress it may become conditionally essential!
It constitutes 60% of free intracellular amino acids in skeletal muscle. Glutamine is the principal metabolic fuel of gut mucosal cells (enterocytes), lymphocytes and monocytes. Recent studies have suggested that addition of glutamine to nutritional regimes may improve outcome in patients with sepsis and after surgery. It is possible that some of the immune dysfunction seen after trauma and sepsis is due to glutamine deficiency.
Coeliac disease is due to allergy to gluten.

Ref: BJA 1996: 177; 118–127.

1.22 Laparoscopic surgery **Answers: A B C D E**

Laparoscopic surgery leads to physiological changes as a result of insufflation of the abdomen with a gas, under pressure, often with the patient in the Trendelenburg position. Thus, the effects of the gas (usually CO_2), include gas embolism, hypercarbia and postoperative shoulder tip pain. The hypercarbia may predispose to arrhythmias and produce an acidosis. The fact that the gas is under pressure predisposes to pneumothorax or pneumomediastinum.

There is reduced thoracic compliance and the airway pressures are elevated. This increases the risk of barotrauma. It also leads to a reduction in functional residual capacity with shunting of blood and hypoxia. The pressure in the peritoneum may be sufficient to reduce venous return, cardiac output and blood pressure. More commonly however, if the patient is in the Trendelenburg position, there is a tachycardia with hypertension.

Intraperitoneal pressure should be monitored and should not exceed 30 cm H_2O. There is an increased risk of regurgitation if the patient is in the Trendelenburg position. Haemorrhage and perforation of a viscus can occur due to damage by the trocar.

1.23 Total hip replacement **Answers: A C**

Total hip replacement can be carried out under regional or general anaesthesia. There is no evidence that regional anaesthesia reduces long-term mortality. Although useful analgesics, NSAIDs may precipitate acute renal failure in the elderly or dehydrated patient. Hyperventilation is of no benefit and in the elderly may cause cerebral vasoconstriction with the risk of stroke. Methyl methacrylate cement may be used in total hip replacement. It is certainly not a positive inotrope.

Intra-operative embolism is not uncommon in this operation and will cause hypoxia. There is usually a tachycardia, hypotension and a sudden drop in end-tidal CO_2 when an embolus occurs.

1.24 Nerve damage in the lithotomy position **Answers: A D**

The lithotomy position may result in nerve damage on the medial or the lateral side of the leg from pressure exerted by the stirrups. The common peroneal (lateral popliteal nerve) may be damaged in this position leading to foot drop, caused by compression of the nerve between the lithotomy pole and the head of the fibula. The saphenous nerve may be damaged if it is trapped between the lithotomy pole and the medial tibial condyle.

Ref: Anaesthesiology 1994: 81; 6–12. Nerve injury after lithotomy.

1.25 Salicylate poisoning **Answers: A B E**

Severe salicylate poisoning can cause profound metabolic upset. The acid-base status of the patient who has taken an aspirin overdose depends on the amount of drug taken. In mild overdose, the patient usually hyperventilates leading to a respiratory alkalosis, as the aspirin directly stimulates the respiratory centre in the brain. In severe aspirin overdose however, there is usually a metabolic acidosis due to uncoupling of oxidative phosphorylation. The blood gases may thus show a mixed respiratory alkalosis and metabolic acidosis.

Hypoprothrombinaemia occurs for which intravenous vitamin K should be given, along with fresh frozen plasma. Thrombocytopenia may occur or there may be impaired platelet function. The serum fibrinogen is normal, and haemolysis does not occur. There may be gastrointestinal bleeding as a result of the coagulopathy.

1.26 Acute Respiratory Distress Syndrome (ARDS) **Answers: A C E**

ARDS is characterised by refractory hypoxia ($PaO_2 < 10$ kPa; $FiO_2 >$ 0.5), with bilateral diffuse pulmonary infiltrates on the CXR, a pulmonary artery wedge pressure of < 18 mmHg (i.e. excluding heart failure or fluid overload as causes) in the context of a recognised risk factor for the development of the syndrome.

The lung compliance is markedly reduced. Thus in a patient with ARDS there is hypoxia, hypercarbia, reduced lung compliance, increased airway resistance and reduced diffusion capacity.

Ref: BMJ 1993: 307; 1335-1339.

1.27 Isoprenaline **Answer: D**

Isoprenaline produces a tachycardia by stimulating beta-1 adrenergic receptors in the heart. Its action may thus be blocked by the beta-blocking drug, propanolol.

Trimetaphan is a ganglion-blocking drug used to reduce blood pressure, which usually results in a compensatory tachycardia.

Atropine is vagolytic, used to treat bradycardia, and will thus exacerbate any tachycardia caused by isoprenaline.

Nifedipine is a calcium-channel-blocking drug used to reduce blood pressure. It usually produces a reflex tachycardia Phentolamine is an antagonist at alpha-1 adrenoreceptors, and when used to treat hypertension can cause a dramatic tachycardia.

1.28 Hepatitis B transmission **Answers: A B D E**

The risk of transmission of hepatitis B has been reduced over the years by careful screening of all blood donors for hepatitis B sAg. Despite this there remains a small risk of viral transmission unless the blood products are pasteurised, heat treated, or treated by some other virucidal procedure. Thus hepatitis B may be transmitted by platelets, packed red cells, plasma (FFP), fibrinogen and cryoprecipitate and human factor VIII. Factor VIII produced by recombinant DNA technology is totally free of risk as regards hepatitis B transmission.

1.29 Anaphylaxis **Answers: A E**

The Association of Anaesthetists of Great Britain & Ireland produced guidelines on the management of suspected anaphylactic reactions associated with anaesthesia in 1995.

Initial therapy:

a) stop administration of drug(s) likely to have caused the anaphylaxis
b) maintain airway; give 100% oxygen
c) lay patient flat with feet elevated
d) give adrenaline
e) start intravascular volume expansion with crystalloid or colloid.

Chlorpheniramine and hydrocortisone are second-line drugs.

1.30 The femoral nerve **Answers: A D E**

The femoral nerve is derived from the anterior primary rami of L2, L3 and L4, and is the largest nerve of the lumbar plexus. It enters the thigh beneath the inguinal ligament and lies 1 cm lateral to the femoral artery, outside the femoral sheath. A 3 in 1 block is a femoral nerve block with a large volume of local anaesthetic (20–30 ml) which diffuses within a single musculo-fascial plane to block the obturator and lateral cutaneous nerve of the thigh.

1.31 Hypotension after removal of a phaeochromocytoma **Answers: A B C D E**

Hypotension after removal of a phaeochromocytoma may be due to all the above causes and in addition may be the result of acute adrenal failure, left ventricular dysfunction or haemorrhage.

1.32 Side-effects of amiodarone **Answers: A B C D E**

Amiodarone is a class III anti-arrhythmic in the Vaughan Williams classification of anti-arrhythmic agents. It is used to treat both ventricular and supraventricular arrhythmias. It has a number of side-effects;

amongst the more benign are a photosensitive grey discolouration to the skin and reversible corneal micro-deposits. Amiodarone is an iodine-containing compound and it therefore can interfere with the thyroid gland. It can produce hypo- and hyperthyroidism. It can lead to potentially fatal pulmonary fibrosis, can cause hepatic dysfunction, and very rarely may cause a peripheral neuropathy.

1.33 Acute tubular necrosis **Answers: D E**

Acute tubular necrosis (ATN) is characterised by:

a) a high urinary sodium concentration (> 40 mEq/l)
b) low urinary urea and creatinine concentrations
c) low urinary osmolality (< 350 mOsm)

In other words, in ATN there is loss of renal concentrating ability by the renal tubules. Thus there is production of poor quality urine with a low osmolality. The tubules fail to conserve sodium and fail to excrete urea and creatinine. By contrast, in dehydration and other causes of pre-renal acute renal failure, the urine is concentrated (urinary osmolality > 400 mosmol/kg), the urinary sodium is low (< 20 mEq/l), and there is a high urinary urea and creatinine.

In ATN there will also be hyperkalaemia, an elevated plasma urea and creatinine, and there may be a rapidly rising CVP with pulmonary oedema.

1.34 Blood gases in aspirin poisoning **Answers: A B C D**

The question is a little ambiguous!

In aspirin overdose there may be:

a) respiratory alkalosis
b) metabolic acidosis
c) a mixed respiratory alkalosis and metabolic acidosis

Salicylates, by stimulating the respiratory system directly, initially cause respiratory alkalosis. However, in overdosage they uncouple oxidative phosphorylation; consequent impairment of aerobic pathways superimposes a metabolic (lactic) acidosis on the respiratory alkalosis. Both respiratory alkalosis and metabolic acidosis result in low blood bicarbonate, but the pH may be high if respiratory alkalosis is predominant, normal if the two cancel each other out, or low if metabolic acidosis is predominant.

Thus a pH of 6.9 is possible, but indicates a very severe overdose. Equally a $PaCO_2$ of 3.2 kPa would be possible, due to respiratory alkalosis. A PaO_2 of 10 kPa is a normal figure for a healthy young adult breathing room air; there is no reason for the PaO_2 to be deranged in salicylate poisoning.

1.35 Nitric oxide **Answers: C E**

Nitric oxide (NO) is a widespread biological mediator. It is synthesised from L-arginine by NO synthases, of which there are three types: endothelial (constitutive), neuronal, and macrophage (inducible). NO is a highly reactive free radical with a half-life of a few seconds.

NO was formerly known as endothelin derived relaxant factor (EDRF). As the name implies it has a pivotal role in the maintenance of vascular tone in both the pulmonary and peripheral circulations. It inhibits platelet aggregation and is a vasodilator.

NO stimulates guanylate cyclase leading to increased formation of cyclic GMP, which then acts at the cellular level to cause vasodilatation, as well as many other effects.

NO is the final pathway for the action of glyceryl trinitrate and other nitrovasodilators.

NO is one of the mediators in the sepsis syndrome causing peripheral vasodilatation. In very low concentrations (around 100 parts per billion) nitric oxide gas has been used to cause selective pulmonary vasodilatation and improve oxygenation. Paradoxically, perhaps, inhibitors of NO synthase such as L-NMMA (NG-monomethyl L-arginine) have been used to correct the peripheral circulatory failure seen in sepsis syndrome.

NO is also a peripheral and central neurotransmitter at nitrergic neurones. It may play a part in the pathogenesis of such diverse conditions as diabetes mellitus, atherosclerosis, hypertension, Alzheimer's disease, Parkinson's disease and stroke.

Ref: BJA 1996: 76; 177–178.

1.36 Spinal block contraindications **Answers: A B C**

None of the above are absolute contraindications to spinal block. However, it is generally accepted that a spinal block can cause marked hypotension consequent upon the autonomic block that it produces. If there is existing hypovolaemia or the likelihood of significant blood loss (e.g. placenta praevia), a spinal block might lead to catastrophic hypotension, and thus it is a relative contraindication to its use in these instances. Although a regional technique is preferable to a general anaesthetic in pre-eclampsia, as it avoids the surge in blood pressure seen with laryngoscopy and intubation, an epidural is preferred to a spinal block as it is less likely to cause profound hypotension.

A breech presentation and fetal distress are not contraindications to a spinal block.

1.37 Tourniquets and nerve damage **Answers: C D E**

Nerve damage from a tourniquet will produce signs of lower motor neurone damage. An extensor plantar response occurs in upper motor neurone damage. If there is nerve damage following the application of a tourniquet to the leg for two hours the ankle jerk may be depressed. There will be reduced pin prick at the toe and reduced vibration sense at the ankle. Stimulation of the common peroneal nerve will produce reduced movement at the ankle.

The Medical Defence Union recently produced an article concerning litigation following damage from tourniquets and made the following recommendations:

a) apply only to healthy limbs
b) tourniquet size: arm 10 cm, leg 15 cm or wider in larger legs
c) pressure: 50–100 mmHg above systolic for the arm; double systolic for the thigh
   OR
   arm 200–250 mmHg, leg 250–350 mmHg
d) time: absolute maximum 3 hours (recovers in 5–7 days); generally do not exceed 2 hours
e) documentation: duration and pressure at the least.

1.38 Immediate problems post-thyroidectomy **Answers: B C D E**

Problems in the postoperative period following a thyroidectomy may be immediate or occur once the patient is back on the ward. Amongst the immediate complications is wound haematoma. The surgeon will usually close the thyroidectomy scar with either clips or staples, and the patient is nursed with a set of instruments at the bedside should it be necessary quickly to evacuate a haematoma which otherwise might lead to tracheal compression and respiratory embarrassment.

Another immediate complication that can occur is tracheal collapse. Hypocalcaemia, due to removal of one or more of the parathyroid glands at surgery, tends to occur in the early postoperative period, but not immediately. Thyroid crisis can occur intra-operatively or at any time in the post-operative period.

Untreated it may result in coma and be fatal. It usually presents with tachycardia, pyrexia, confusion and abdominal pain and requires treatment with beta blockers and anti-thyroid drugs. Laryngeal stridor may occur due to oedema or direct damage to one or both of the recurrent laryngeal nerves.

1.39 Hypertensive drug interaction with MAOIs **Answers: A D**

Patients taking monoamine oxidase inhibitors as treatment for depression can develop severe hypertensive crises due to an interaction with ephedrine. The appropriate treatment for such a reaction includes using vasodilators to reverse the intense peripheral vasoconstriction responsible for the hypertension. Thus labetalol, phentolamine and diazoxide would all be of use in this situation.

1.40 Extrapyramidal side-effects **Answers: C D E**

Any drug which is an antagonist at dopaminergic receptors can produce extrapyramidal side-effects. In this respect perphenazine is one of the drugs most likely to cause problems. Droperidol also commonly causes this side-effect. The range of extrapyramidal side-effects includes Parkinsonism, dystonia (facial grimacing), akathisia (restlessness) and tardive dyskinesia.

Treatment includes withdrawal of the drug, and administration of an antimuscarinic drug such as procyclidine or benztropine.

1.41 Propranolol **Answer: C**

Propranolol is a non-selective beta blocker, with actions at both beta-1 and beta-2 adrenoceptors. It causes an increase in airways resistance by blockade of beta-2 receptors in the lungs. Beta blockers are contraindicated with verapamil as they are both negative inotropes. In particular, intravenous verapamil can lead to hypotension and asystole if given to a patient on beta blockers. Beta blockers can lead to a small deterioration in glucose tolerance in diabetics, as well as, more importantly, masking the signs of hypoglycaemia. In the non-diabetic, beta blockers do not cause hyperglycaemia.

1.42 Epidural analgesia **Answers: A B D**

It is accepted that epidural analgesia may lead to both a prolonged second stage of labour and an increased rate of instrumental delivery. What remains a disputed issue is whether there is an increased rate of caesarian section in parturients who recieve epidural analgesia. The evidence to date suggests that there is no association between backache post-partum and the siting of an epidural. Both urinary retention and headache are potential complications of epidurals. The latter is due to inadvertent puncture of the dura and may require an epidural blood patch to treat it. There is a reduced rate of deep vein thrombosis with epidural anaesthesia.

Ref: BJA; Feb 1997: 78; 115–117.
Ref: Fetal & Maternal Medicine Review 1996: 8; 29–55.

1.43 Features of Down's syndrome **Answers: A B C E**

Down's syndrome is due to trisomy of chromosome 21. It occurs in about 1 in 1000 live births; meiotic non-dysjunction is responsible for 90% of cases and is related to maternal age. There is a characteristic facies with a flat face, slanting eyes and epicanthic folds. There may be a single transverse palmar crease. A webbed neck occurs in Turner's syndrome (45 XO).
Down's syndrome is associated with congenital heart disease, which occurs in about 40% of cases. These include Tetralogy of Fallot (10%), patent ductus arteriosus (10%), ventricular septal defect (25%), atrial septal defect and endocardial cushion defects (40%).

The following are also features of, or occur more commonly in Down's syndrome: acute lymphoblastic leukaemia, mental impairment, cataracts, epilepsy, scoliosis, duodenal atresia.

The anaesthetic implications mainly concern the airway. Intubation may be difficult due to a big tongue and small mouth. Atlanto-axial subluxation with instability occurs in about 15%. Sub-glottic stenosis may occur, necessitating an endotracheal tube of a smaller diameter than usual.

1.44 Features of bronchial carcinoma **Answers: A C D E**

Carcinoma of the bronchus most commonly presents with haemoptysis and weight loss in a heavy smoker. The prognosis is poor, unless the tumour is localised and resectable. Most tumours respond poorly to either chemo- or radiotherapy, and many have metastasised to bone or other organs at the time of diagnosis. A patient with a Pancoast tumour in the apex of the lung invading the brachial plexus may present with Horner's syndrome.

There are many non-metastatic paraneoplastic syndromes that can occur in lung cancer including autonomic neuropathy, cerebellar degeneration, peripheral neuropathy and Eaton-Lambert syndrome. In about 10% of tumours there may be production of ectopic hormones such as ADH or parathormone. Clubbing and hypertrophic pulmonary osteoarthropathy can occur. Although not common, a lymphocytic meningitis can occur.

1.45 Pulmonary artery occlusion pressure **Answer: All false**

The pulmonary artery occlusion pressure (PAOP) is measured with a flow-directed pulmonary artery catheter. Assuming that there is an uninterrupted column of blood from the pulmonary artery to the left atrium then the PAOP should be an accurate reflection of left atrial pressure (LAP). As long as there is no pressure gradient across the mitral valve then LAP should = left ventricular end diastolic pressure (LVEDP). The final assumption in the measurement of PAOP is that, in the normally compliant left ventricle LVEDP = left ventricular end diastolic volume.

Thus measurement of PAOP assumes that: PAOP=LAP=LVEDP=LVEDV. This does not always hold true. In myocardial infarction, cardiomyopathy and severe aortic regurgitation the compliance of the left ventricle is reduced and LVEDP does not equate with LVEDV. In mitral stenosis the LAP is elevated and so PAOP/LAP does not reflect LVEDP.

1.46 Prognostic indicators in ITU **Answers: C E**

The prognosis for a group of patients admitted to ITU with a specific diagnosis is based on the APACHE 3 scoring system. APACHE stands for acute physiology and chronic health evaluation. In the original APACHE 1 there were 34 physiological variables. This was reduced to 12 in APACHE 2. APACHE 3 included a further 6 variables.

The 12 variables in APACHE 2 are: rectal temperature, mean arterial pressure, heart rate, respiratory rate, arterial pH, arterial PaO_2, serum sodium, potassium and creatinine, haematocrit, white cell count and Glasgow coma scale.

1.47 Endotoxin **Answers: B D E**

Endotoxin is the part of a micro-organism which if present in sufficient amounts in the bloodstream will lead to the development of the sepsis syndrome, characterised by peripheral circulatory failure with systemic hypotension, pulmonary hypertension, pyrexia, tachycardia and either leucopenia or a neutrophil leucocytosis. Endotoxin is not invariably found in septic patients, but the test for its presence does use crabs blood!
The presence of endotoxin is thought to lead to the production of cytokines and other inflammatory mediators. In particular nitric oxide (NO) and the cytokines interleukin-6 (IL-6) and tumour necrosis factor-alpha (TNF) are thought to play an important part in the pathogenesis of the sepsis syndrome.
Although no longer available, an antibody directed against the A antigen of endotoxin was used as a treatment for sepsis. A trial looking at the efficacy of using this monoclonal antibody (called HA-1A, Centoxin) in patients with Gram-negative septicaemia was suspended.

1.48 Estimate of cardiac output **Answers: B E**

There has been much controversy recently concerning the use of pulmonary artery (PA) catheters. A recent study in the *Journal of the American Medical Association* (JAMA) suggested that inserting a PA catheter led to an increased mortality in ITU patients and the authors asked the FDA to put a moratorium on the use of PA catheters, pending a prospective, double-blind, randomised study.

Ref: BMJ 1996: 313; 763–764.
Ref: JAMA 1996: 276(11); 889–898.
Ref: NEJM 1995: 333(16); 1025–1031.

1.49 The ECG **Answers: All false**

In the ECG the P wave represents atrial depolarisation and the T wave ventricular repolarisation. The QRS complex represents ventricular depolarisation. A positive deflection occurs when the depolarisation is going towards the recording electrode. Sodium is the major ion causing the transmembrane potential. There are six recording V electrodes. The duration of the QRS complex is constant, no matter which lead it is recorded from.

1.50 Adequacy of perfusion in posterior fossa surgery Answers: B C E

If perfusion is reduced in posterior fossa surgery there is usually a rise in blood pressure (Cushing's reflex) in an attempt to compensate. There is often an associated bradycardia or arrhythmias and an abnormal respiratory pattern. Delta waves on the EEG are non-specific as the EEG is affected by so many other variables including the anaesthetic agents.

1.51 Propofol Answers: A C D

Propofol is 2,6 di-isopropyl phenol. It is presented in a 1% solution (10 mg/ml) as a white emulsion containing soybean oil, egg phosphatide and glycerol. It is a rapidly acting intravenous anaesthetic agent with a rapid, clear recovery. It is metabolised mainly in the liver, but also in extrahepatic sites such as the lungs.

In terms of side-effects, it causes a 15–25% drop in blood pressure by a reduction in cardiac output and systemic vascular resistance, which is of greater magnitude than that seen with thiopentone. It causes pain on injection and can cause green discolouration of the urine. It is not licensed for use in patients under the age of 3 years. It is safe in patients with malignant hyperpyrexia and in porphyria and patients with egg allergy, but should be avoided in patients with disorders of fat metabolism.

It has an anti-emetic action and in the CNS causes a reduction in cerebral blood flow, metabolism and intracranial pressure. It depresses laryngeal reflexes such that laryngeal mask insertion is facilitated and laryngospasm is uncommon.

1.52 Wright's respirometer Answers: A B D

The Wright respirometer, a turbine, measures gas volume (e.g. tidal or minute volume). It under-reads at < 1 l/min and is affected by moisture which causes the pointer to stick. The pneumotachograph measures flow rate (e.g. peak flow). It is affected by gas viscosity.

1.53 Nitrous oxide Answers: A C E

Nitrous oxide (N_2O) is a colourless gas which is stored in French blue cylinders as a liquid at a pressure of 54 bar. Nitrous oxide affects vitamin B12 synthesis by inhibiting the enzyme methionine synthetase. Exposure to nitrous oxide for 6 hours or longer may result in megaloblastic anaemia. Nitrous oxide also interferes with folic acid metabolism. Because nitrous oxide is 35 times more soluble in blood than nitrogen, it will diffuse into air filled cavities, such as the middle ear, faster than the nitrogen diffuses out. Thus the pressure in the middle ear will increase and therefore in tympanoplasty nitrous oxide is a relative contra-indication.

1.54 A fixed low cardiac output state **Answers: C E**

A fixed low cardiac output state occurs in constrictive pericarditis and aortic stenosis. In anaemia there is a compensatory increase in cardiac output to maintain tissue oxygen delivery.

In Paget's disease there is often high output cardiac failure. The abnormal bone has such a huge vasculature that it puts great demands on the myocardium and the cardiac output is increased to such an extent as to cause the heart to fail.

Eisenmenger's syndrome occurs when pulmonary hypertension develops in the context of a long-standing ventricular septal defect. The result is a reversal of the shunt so that the shunt becomes right to left. This results in an elevated cardiac output.

1.55 Emphysema and chronic bronchitis **Answer: E**

The classical 'pink puffer', when compared with the 'blue bloater', retains the drive to respiration that CO_2 produces on the central medullary respiratory centre. Thus the 'pink puffer' has a lower $PaCO_2$ and a higher PaO_2, compared to the 'blue bloater'.

Because the 'blue bloater' tends to be hypoxic, he has a higher haematocrit (secondary polycythaemia usually occurs). The hypoxia of the 'blue bloater' leads to pulmonary hypertension and cor pulmonale.

In reality the 'pink puffer' and 'blue bloater' represent two ends of a spectrum in chronic obstructive airways disease, and most patients have characteristics of both.

1.56 Obesity **Answers: B E**

Obesity is a metabolic disease in which adipose tissue comprises a greater proportion of body tissue than normal. Obesity predisposes to ischaemic heart disease, hypertension and diabetes mellitus. Hiatus hernia is more common, predisposing to regurgitation of acidic stomach contents and subsequent pneumonitis. In addition there is a greater incidence of difficult intubation in the obese. Chest wall and lung compliance is reduced. The functional residual capacity (FRC) is reduced and falls further with anaesthesia causing the closing volume to encroach on the FRC during normal tidal ventilation. This leads to increased V/Q mismatch and hypoxaemia due to the large intrapulmonary shunt. The incidence of thromboembolic problems such as deep vein thrombosis and pulmonary embolus is increased and so obese patients should be given prophylactic heparin prior to anything except minor surgery. Venous access and regional blocks may be technically difficult, as may finding an adequately sized blood pressure cuff.

Ref: BJA 1993: 70; 349–359.

1.57 Peak flow **Answers: B C D E**

Peak flow is measured by the pneumotachograph. It is reduced in an acute attack of asthma and may be used to monitor the response to therapy. There is a diurnal variation in peak flow, caused by the diurnal variation in cortisol levels, which are lowest in early morning. This may cause morning dipping and episodes of wheezing in asthmatics. The measurement of peak flow is very operator dependent, and may be artefactually low in weak and debilitated patients.

1.58 Flail chest **Answers: C D**

In a patient with flail chest, being ventilated and losing 1.5 l/min, treatment might include increasing fresh gas flow by 1.5 l/min and reducing peak inspiratory flow rate.

1.59 In a pressure generator ventilator **Answers: B C**

A pressure generator ventilator produces a constant pressure by bellows or a weight. An example is the Manley ventilator. Although this is a minute volume divider, not all pressure generators are. Cycling from inspiration to expiration, and vice versa, may be time cycled. Barotrauma is more of a risk in pressure generators compared with constant flow generators.

1.60 Paracetamol poisoning **Answers: A B D E**

The most serious problem with paracetamol overdose is hepatotoxicity. This is due to a toxic metabolite of paracetamol metabolism by the liver, which is normally scavenged by intracellular glutathione. In overdose the supply of glutathione is exhausted and the toxic metabolite then causes hepatocellullar centrilobular necrosis. N-acetylcysteine and methionine will act to mop up the toxic metabolite and prevent hepatic damage.

The hepatic damage, if it occurs, is not apparent until 48 hours after the overdose. It causes a rise in the liver enzymes and a prolongation of the prothrombin time. The prothrombin time may be used to assess the degree of liver damage and may also be of prognostic value. In the most severe cases fulminant hepatic necrosis may occur, and liver transplant may be necessary.

1.61 Brachial plexus blocks **Answers: A C E**

A supraclavicular brachial plexus block is more likely to produce side-effects than an axillary block. Supraclavicular blocks can be complicated by:

a) pneumothorax
b) intravascular injection
c) phrenic nerve block
d) Horner's syndrome

Apart from intravascular injection, the axillary approach to the brachial plexus is relatively free of complications. The supraclavicular approach, however, produces the most complete anaesthesia of the brachial plexus.

1.62 Autonomic nervous system **Answers: A B C D**

The autonomic nervous system consists of the sympathetic and parasympathetic systems. Acetylcholine is the neurotransmitter at all ganglia, at post-ganglionic parasympathetic nerves, and at the sympathetic nerves innervating the sweat glands.

Noradrenaline is the neurotransmitter at post-ganglionic sympathetic nerves. Whilst the action of acetylcholine is mainly terminated by metabolism, that of noradrenaline is mainly terminated by re-uptake into the nerve terminal.

The noradrenaline produced by sympathetic nerve endings acts on cell surface receptors of either alpha or beta type. Activation of beta receptors leads in turn to activation of the enzyme adenylate cyclase. Beta-2 receptors are found in the uterus and their stimulation results in relaxation of the uterus.

1.63 Pre-eclampsia **Answers: A B**

Severe pre-eclampsia implies organ damage: blood pressure of 160/110 mmHg or greater at rest, severe proteinuria and oliguria, and central nervous system irritability, with headaches and visual problems. Magnesium sulphate is now the anticonvulsant of choice. Magnesium is both a membrane stabiliser and a vasodilator, so improving placental blood flow. Thrombocytopenia is the most common haematological abnormality seen in severe pre-eclampsia. The HELLP syndrome (Haemolysis, Elevated Liver function tests, and Low Platelets), is a form of severe pre-eclampsia. Both the prothrombin and partial thrombo-plastin times are usually normal and DIC is very rare. The parturient with severe pre-eclampsia is usually advised to have a caesarean section. A regional, rather than general anaesthesia, is the preferred mode of anaesthesia as it avoids the pressor response to laryngoscopy and intubation. Although these women are often oedematous they have, nevertheless, a contracted intravascular volume. They thus require intravenous fluids in conjunction with close monitoring of urine output and central venous pressure. The aim is to avoid fluid overload and pulmonary oedema, while ensuring an adequate urine output to prevent acute renal failure.

Ref: The Lancet 1995: 345; 1455–1463.

1.64 Penicillins **Answer: B**

The penicillins are bactericidal and act by interfering with bacterial cell wall synthesis. The most important side-effect of the penicillins is hypersensitivity, which causes rashes and, occasionally, anaphylaxis, which can be fatal. 10% of patients who are allergic to penicillins will also be allergic to cephalosporins.

The penicillins are active against both Gram-positive and Gram-negative organisms. It would be unusual to choose a penicillin as first-line treatment for a UTI; the commonest cause for UTI is *E. coli* for which trimethoprim is the first-choice antibiotic.

1.65 Glycosuria **Answers: A B C D E**

Glycosuria occurs in diabetes mellitus and any cause of secondary diabetes such as acromegaly, phaeochromocytoma, Cushing's syndrome, steroid therapy, thiazides and haemochromatosis. Glycosuria occurs in pregnancy, following partial gastrectomy and pancreatectomy, and may occur following head injury as part of the body's general stress response.

1.66 Chronic renal failure **Answers: A B C D E**

This topic was covered in answer 1.9. Chronic renal failure causes a normochromic, normocytic anaemia. Patients have hypergastrinaemia gastric erosions and may therefore have an iron deficiency anaemia. It may be secondary to or cause hypertension. It causes defective platelet function and a bleeding diathesis as a result. As a result of the metabolic acidosis of renal failure there is a right shift of the oxygen-haemoglobin dissociation curve. The hypocalcaemia of chronic renal failure induces secondary hyperparathyroidism.

1.67 Contraindications to suxamethonium **Answers: A C**

This topic was discussed in answer 1.20. There is no contraindication to the use of suxamethonium in porphyria. It is, however, a potent trigger for malignant hyperpyrexia, the other inherited condition that is of particular relevance to anaesthetists. It is contraindicated in dystrophia myotonica, where its administration may lead to such severe masseter muscle spasm as to render intubation impossible.

In acute renal failure there is hyperkalaemia. Since suxamethonium leads to a rise in serum potassium of up to 0.5–1.0 mmol/l, its administration in renal failure may precipitate cardiac arrest from ventricular fibrillation.

There is no evidence to suggest that suxamethonium is contraindicated in Creutzfelt-Jakob disease.

Following spinal cord injury suxamethonium is indeed contraindicated, but the dangerous rise in serum potassium that its administration may cause in this situation does not occur until several days after the spinal injury.

1.68 Thyroid storm **Answers: A B C D E**

Thyroid storm is the term given to a condition resembling acute thyrotoxicosis, occurring soon after a partial thyroidectomy. Signs include pyrexia (for which paracetamol may be given), flushing and sweating. There is usually a tachycardia, sometimes atrial fibrillation and high output cardiac failure. Propanolol, verapamil and digoxin may be used to treat the cardiac problems. Patients are often confused, restless or delirious and require sedation with a benzodiazepine or anti-psychotic medication such as chlorpromazine. In addition, the patients may require active cooling, rehydration with intravenous fluids, supplementary oxygen and antithyroid medication.

1.69 Porphyrias **Answers: B D E**

The porphyrias are a group of inherited metabolic diseases in which there is an abnormality of porphyrin metabolism. Haem of haemoglobin contains a central porphyrin ring. If abnormally metabolised the porphyric patient may suffer an acute attack, which may be precipitated by a number of drugs including, classically, the barbiturates such as thiopentone or methohexitone. Pancuronium is not safe, but propofol and all the volatile agents are. In addition all the local anaesthetic agents are safe: thus a regional technique should be employed where possible.

Ref: Anaesthesia 1993: 48; 417–421.
Ref: Current Anaesthesia & Critical Care 1996: 7; 37–43.

1.70 Thrombolytic therapy **Answers: C E**

Thrombolytic therapy is given to treat acute myocardial infarction. Streptokinase, tissue-type plasminogen activator (rt-PA) and APSAC (anistreplase) are the three commonly available thrombolytic agents. No one agent has been shown to be superior to the others.

Aspirin has an additive effect when combined with streptokinase in terms of reducing mortality. Thrombolytic therapy is contraindicated if there has been recent surgery, trauma or haemorrhage. Streptokinase cannot be given for a second time within three months of the previous dose, because of the risk of serious allergic reactions.

Malignant ventricular arrhythmias are very rare, but so called reperfusion arrhythmias do occur following thrombolytic therapy.

1.71 Sensory signs **Answers: A B C E**

Motor neurone disease, as the name implies, affects only motor neurones and there are no sensory signs.

In multiple sclerosis there are often sensory symptoms and signs. It may present with retro bulbar neuritis or paraesthesia and numbness in a limb.

Carpal tunnel syndrome is due to compression of the median nerve at the wrist as it passes deep to the flexor retinaculum. It produces pain and sensory signs in the distribution of the median nerve in the hand.

Tabes dorsalis is caused by tertiary syphilis and presents with signs of damage to the dorsal columns of the spinal cord, such as ataxia.

Syringomyelia is caused by an expanding cavity within the spinal cord which causes loss of pain and temperature sensation in the arms.

1.72 Fixed cardiac output state **Answers: A B D E**

In both aortic stenosis and hypertrophic obstructive cardiomyopathy (HOCM), there is obstruction to the outflow from the left ventricle either at the level of the valve or sub-valvular. This results in a fixed, low cardiac output state.

In mitral stenosis there is also a fixed low cardiac output state as there is obstruction to the passage of blood from the left atrium to the left ventricle through the mitral valve.

In constrictive pericarditis the ventricles cannot relax fully in diastole so that ventricular filling is inadequate and the cardiac output is therefore low and also fixed.

In persistent ductus arteriosus (PDA), by contrast, there is a hyperdynamic circulation with a collapsing pulse and a high cardiac output as there is a connection between the aorta and the pulmonary artery.

1.73 Phantom limb pain **Answers: A B**

Phantom limb pain is difficult to treat. It may be worsened by spinal anaesthesia but may be improved by establishing an epidural block prior to amputation. Opioids are generally ineffective in phantom limb pain.

1.74 A retrobulbar block **Answers: A C E**

Local eye blocks are of two main sorts: retrobulbar and peribulbar. In a retrobulbar block, local anaesthetic is injected within the muscle cone around the orbit, whereas in a peribulbar block the injection is outside the muscle cone. Within the muscle cone lie the optic, oculomotor, abducent and nasociliary (short and long ciliary) nerves. Thus all these nerves, except the optic nerve (which has a dural sheath), are blocked in a retrobulbar block.

With a retrobulbar block a separate facial nerve block is required and orbital akinesia is produced within 5 minutes.

A peribulbar block takes longer (15–30 mins) and requires a greater volume of local anaesthetic, but may be associated with fewer serious complications, such as perforation of the globe. A separate facial nerve block is unnecessary.

Ref: British Journal of Hospital Medicine 1993: 49(10); 689–701.
Ref: BJA 1995: 75; 80–87.

1.75 Sensory innervation of the hand **Answers: A B**

The sensation of the palm of the hand is supplied by the median and ulnar nerves. The median nerve supplies sensation to the thenar eminence and the palmar aspect of the radial three and a half digits, while the ulnar nerve supplies sensation to the rest of the palmar surface of the hand.

1.76 Treatments for poisoning **Answer: D**

Oral methionine, or, more usually, intravenous N-acetylcysteine is used to treat paracetamol poisoning. Coma and respiratory failure are unusual in salicylate poisoning and assisted ventilation is thus rare. Dicobalt edetate is used as an antidote in cyanide poisoning.

Physostigmine may be used as a last resort in severe tricyclic overdose, where anti-arrhythmic agents have failed, but it may cause seizures, bradycardia and cardiac failure, and therefore is not generally recommended.

1.77 Apgar score **Answers: A B D**

Dr Virginia Apgar, an American anaesthetist, designed a simple scoring system to assess neonatal well being. Scores of 0, 1 or 2 are given to each of the following five variables:

a) heart rate
b) respiratory effect
c) muscle tone
d) reflex movement
e) colour

A score out of 10 is reached, having been measured at 1 and 5 minutes after delivery of the baby's head.

1.78 Nerves to block for mid-thigh amputation **Answers: A C**

To provide adequate analgesia for a mid-thigh amputation one would need to block the femoral lateral cutaneous nerve of the thigh and the posterior cutaneous nerve of the thigh. The cutaneous branches of the anterior division of the femoral nerve supply sensation to the skin over the antero-medial part of the thigh.

The lateral cutaneous nerve of the thigh supplies sensation to the anterolateral part of the thigh, and the posterior cutaneous nerve of the thigh, not surprisingly, supplies sensation to the posterior part of the thigh.

The sciatic nerve provides the innervation of the calf and the foot, while the obturator nerve supplies sensation to the hip and knee joints.

1.79 Anti-dopaminergic drugs **Answer: E**

Dopaminergic receptors are subdivided into DA1 and DA2 receptors. In the CNS, DA1 receptors affect extrapyramidal activity and their blockade can produce Parkinsonism.

DA2 receptors in the CNS affect pituitary hormone release. Blockade of these receptors can produce hyperprolactinaemia and galactorrhoea. Their stimulation by bromocriptine is used to treat acromegaly and hyperprolactinaemia.

DA1 receptors at the chemoreceptor trigger zone mediate emesis and their blockade is the mode of action of many anti-emetics.

Outside the CNS, DA1 receptor stimulation relaxes smooth muscle in the gut and renal vasculature. Antagonism at these receptors promotes gastric emptying and reduces oesophageal reflux. Clinically, however, there is little effect on renal blood flow, and no effect on the coronary circulation.

1.80 Weaning from mechanical ventilation **Answers: C**

About 20% of all ventilated patients fail to be weaned initially. There are many reasons why such patients fail to wean. Impaired respiratory muscle strength may be due to malnutrition, acidosis, hypoxia or hypomagnesaemia, hypophosphataemia or hypocalcaemia. Factors such as bronchospasm or pulmonary oedema increase the load on the respiratory muscles and make successful weaning unlikely. The level of consciousness is important, and patients who are sedated are unlikely to wean rapidly. One bedside assessment of respiratory muscle strength is the Pi max. Most adults can achieve –100 cm H_2O. A severely weak patient might generate a Pi max of –20 cm H_2O. A Pi max of –30 cm H_2O suggests that a patient might wean.

Ref: Current Anaesthesia & Critical Care. 1996: 7; 37–43.

1.81 Aortic regurgitation **Answer: E**

In aortic regurgitation patients complain of dyspnoea, palpitations, chest pain (in the absence of coronary atheroma), and dizziness. Although the stroke volume is increased it is not a threefold increase. The murmur is an early blowing diastolic murmur, maximal on held expiration, sitting forward and in the 3rd or 4th intercostal space. There may be an associated diastolic thrill. The pressure gradient across the valve is in diastole, not systole.

1.82 Mannitol **Answers: B C D E**

Mannitol is an alcohol, not a sugar. It may be used to prevent the hepatorenal syndrome in jaundiced patients. It is found in dantrolene, the specific therapy for malignant hyperpyrexia. It may be used in patients with cerebral oedema. Because it is a hypertonic solution it draws cerebral oedema into the vascular compartment by osmosis. This may lead, however, to circulatory overload. Also, if the blood-brain barrier is damaged and permeable there may be a paradoxical worsening of neurological status after administration of mannitol.

1.83 Pulmonary fibrosis **Answers: A B C E**

The causes of pulmonary fibrosis include the drugs busulphan, bleomycin, cyclophosphamide, nitrofurantoin, amiodarone, beryllium and paraquat, to name but a few. Steroids are sometimes used to treat pulmonary fibrosis. Pulmonary fibrosis is associated with auto-immune and connective tissue diseases and occupational dusts.

1.84 Ulcerative colitis **Answers: A B C D E**

Ulcerative colitis is an inflammatory condition of the colon. It is often accompanied by liver disease ranging from ascending cholangitis to cirrhosis. In long-standing disease there is a significant risk of malignant change. Patients may show clubbing of the fingers. Treatment may involve the use of corticosteroids.

1.85 Obstructive jaundice **Answers: B C**

In obstructive jaundice the patient may complain of pale stools and dark urine. This is because there is no stercobilin in the stools and an elevated amount of conjugated bilirubin in the urine. Because there is obstruction to the passage of bile into the gut there is reduced vitamin K absorption and a resultant coagulopathy. In addition lack of bile salts leads to defective gut absorption of the other fat-soluble vitamins (A, D, E) and of fat itself, leading to steatorrhoea. The stools have a high faecal fat content and therefore tend to float.

Classically, in obstructive jaundice, the alkaline phosphatase and gamma GT are elevated, compared with an elevated AST and ALT in jaundice from hepatocellular damage.

1.86 Negative nitrogen balance **Answers: B C E**

A catabolic state, with associated muscle breakdown and a negative nitrogen balance exists post surgery. It is also found in patients receiving steroids and in starvation. In acute renal failure there is a failure to excrete the nitrogenous waste products of metabolism, and a positive nitrogen balance.

1.87 Intra-operative bronchospasm **Answers: A B D**

Bronchospasm may be precipitated by pharmacological means. Morphine can cause histamine release which may then cause bronchospasm and wheeze. Pethidine has a lesser potential for histamine release, and may be preferred to morphine as a premed in an asthmatic. Atracurium and suxamethonium can also cause histamine release. Neostigmine blocks the action of acetylcholine esterase and therefore is a parasympathomimetic. It may thus cause bronchospasm. Isoflurane, like all the other volatile agents, relaxes bronchial smooth muscle.

Light anaesthesia and stimulation of the trachea or carina by an endotracheal tube may lead to bronchospasm.

1.88 Reticulocytosis **Answers: C E**

A raised reticulocyte count indicates haemolysis. A reticulocytosis will occur once iron deficiency or megaloblastic anaemia is treated. Sickle cell disease, but not the trait, leads to a haemolytic state. Congenital spherocytosis is a hereditary haemolytic disorder.

1.89 Pregnancy **Answers: A D E**

Enormous physiological changes occur in pregnancy. There is an increase in tidal volume and a reduction in FRC, while vital capacity is unchanged. Alveolar ventilation is increased, and the maternal $PaCO_2$ is reduced. Airway resistance is usually unaffected by pregnancy. There is an increase in fibrinogen with reduced fibrinolysis and thus a hyper-coaguable state.

There is an increase in heart rate and stroke volume and thus an elevated cardiac output. A reduction in systemic vascular resistance means that, overall, blood pressure is unchanged (in the absence of pregnancy induced hypertension, which is common). The syndrome of supine hypotension from aorto-caval compression occurs in about 20% of pregnant women from 20 weeks onwards. The blood volume increases about 40% by term: though the increase in plasma volume is greater than the increase in red cell mass, leading to the physiological anaemia of pregnancy.

From the anaesthetic perspective the implications of anaesthetising a pregnant woman depend on the maturity of the fetus. In the first trimester the problems of teratogenicity from the anaesthetic drugs is the major concern. However, there is no evidence that any of the commonly

employed anaesthetic agents are teratogens.
After 20 weeks there may be aorto-caval compression. There is an increased risk of aspiration and difficult intubation in the obstetric population. All mothers undergoing caesarean section receive antacid prophylaxis in the form of a histamine type 2 receptor antagonist and sodium citrate.

1.90 Treatment modalities for ARDS **Answers: A B C D E**

The topic of ARDS was discussed in answer 1.26.
Numerous therapeutic options have been tried in ARDS. Pulmonary hypertension is often present and may be treated using nebulised prostacyclin or inhaled nitric oxide. Ventilatory strategies include pressure control ventilation with inverse I:E ratio, the use of high frequency jet ventilation, IVOX, ECMO ECO2R, and the use of perfluorocarbons.

Ref: BMJ 1993: 307; 1335–1339.

PRACTICE EXAM 1: MODEL VIVA ANSWERS

Viva 1

Examiner 1

Summarise this lady's case.
This is an elderly lady with significant cardiovascular pathology who has refused local anaesthesia. In the past she has suffered a myocardial infarction and an embolus to the right arm.

Clinical examination reveals that she is in atrial fibrillation, with probable mixed mitral valve disease and V and a degree of left ventricular failure.

Current medications are digoxin (for her AF), frumil (for her LVF) and warfarin (previous embolism).

Tell me about her ECG.
You should go systematically through her ECG telling the examiner about the rate, rhythm, axis and any abnormalities.

There are no P waves seen and the rhythm is irregularly irregular. She is in atrial fibrillation. In addition, there is left ventricular hypertrophy. The voltage of the R wave in V1 and S in V5 are greater than 35mm, fulfilling the voltage criteria for LVH.

Describe the CXR.
Again, the examiner will expect you to go through it systematically. Describe the cardiac outline, the lung fields and any obvious pathology. This lady's CXR shows left ventricular hypertrophy and some fine shadowing at the lung bases.

How would you anaesthetise this lady?
She has refused a local eye block, although as she is anticoagulated this is contraindicated anyway.

I would give a general anaesthetic and intubate and ventilate. In order to avoid increased intra-ocular pressure I would maintain normocapnia and avoid venous congestion in the neck veins.

Because of her cardiac history, I would endeavour to avoid changes in blood pressure and heart rate. In particular, with mitral stenosis she may have a relatively fixed cardiac output and would not tolerate changes in heart rate or blood pressure.

Examiner 2

Tell me about premedication.
This involves not only discussing anxiolytes (eg. benzodiazepines) and analgesics (eg. Omnopon) but also antisialagogue (eg. hyoscine), anti-emetics (eg. metaclopramide), EMLA cream, ranitidine, sodium citrate etc.

Tell me about the anaesthetic complications following thyroidectomy.
You need to discuss intra and postoperative problems. The major group of problems are airway problems, such as tracheal collapse, laryngeal nerve palsy causing stridor, and haematomas causing airway compression. You need to discus the management of each of these problems. Haematoma needs to be evacuated urgently. Stridor may require re-intubation which should be done as a controlled gaseous induction technique by an experienced anaesthetist.

How would you anaesthetise a 25-year-old asthmatic who has a blood pressure of 170/100 and is due to have an inguinal hernia repair?
The answer in simple terms is to defer the operation until the hypertension is controlled.

Viva 2: Model Answers

Examiner 1

Tell me about the anaemia of chronic renal failure.
In chronic renal failure, there is usually a normochromic, normocytic anaemia. This is due to reduced production of erythropoietin by the kidneys. As a compensatory mechanism to ensure adequate tissue oxygenation the oxygen-haemoglobin dissociation curve shifts to the right. This is facilitated by the metabolic acidosis that occurs and an increase in 2,3 DPG. The anaemia may be corrected by subcutaneous erythropoietin (EPO) produced by recombinant DNA technology, or by transfusion of red blood cells.

Tell me about the causes of delayed gastric emptying.
Factors that may delay gastric emptying include:

Physiological factors
- Food
- Obesity
- Posture
- Pregnancy and labour

Pathological factors
- Anxiety
- Pain
- Shock
- Trauma
- Diabetic autonomic neuropathy
- Myxoedema
- Scleroderma
- Pyloric stenosis
- Electrolyte disturbance

Pharmacological factors
- Opoids
- Anticholinergic drugs
- Alcohol
- Tricyclic antidepressants
- Aluminium hydroxide

Examiner 2

Tell me about the anatomy of the caudal canal.
The caudal space is a continuation of the epidural space. In the adult the spinal cord ends at L 1 / 2. The dural sac terminates at the level of the second sacral vertebra. Below this is the caudal space.

Failure of fusion of the laminae of the fifth sacral vertebra produces the sacral hiatus; a horseshoe shaped indentation bounded laterally by the sacral cornua. Access to the space is via the sacrococcygeal membrane.

The caudal space contains veins, fat and the sacral nerve roots including S2, S3 and S4, which carry parasympathetic fibres and innervate the uterus and bladder.

Tell me about the problems of hypotensive anaesthesia.
Hypotensive anaesthesia is employed to reduce blood loss and to facilitate visualisation of the surgical field in ENT, orthopaedic and microsurgical operations.

Contraindications include hypertension, ischaemic or valvular heart disease or a previous stroke. Hypovolaemia, pregnancy, anaemia, renal and hepatic disease are relative contraindications.

The problems encountered with hypotensive anaesthesia are due to reduced perfusion of vital organs if the blood pressure falls below the usual autoregulatory threshold.

The cerebral circulation autoregulates blood flow between a mean arterial blood pressure of 50 and 150 mmHg. Cerebral infarction (stroke) may occur in severe hypotension.

Coronary perfusion depends on many factors but in particular requires an adequate diastolic blood pressure. Hypotensive anaesthesia may thus precipitate myocardial ischaemia or infarction.

Renal perfusion ceases below a mean arterial blood pressure of 60 mmHg.

PRACTICE EXAMINATION 2

SHORT ANSWER QUESTION PAPER 2

1. How would you pre-operatively assess, investigate and resuscitate a 6-week-old infant prior to repair of congenital hypertrophic pyloric stenosis?

2. What are the preconditions for testing and how would you perform brain stem death testing?

3. A primigravid woman is found collapsed in the delivery suite following an epidural 'top-up' administered by the midwife 5 minutes earlier. List the likely causes and the initial management.

4. A previously fit 30-year-old male sustains an isolated fracture of the femur during a motor cycle accident. Six hours after admission he becomes dyspnoeic. What are the likely causes and their initial management?

5. Describe your management of an adult patient brought into the accident and emergency department in status epilepticus.

6. How may nutrition be provided for patients on the intensive care unit? What are the advantages and disadvantages of each?

7. What are the indications for awake intubation in the adult? How may the airway be anaesthetised prior to intubation?

8. How may gas exchange and anaesthesia be maintained during rigid bronchoscopy? What problems are associated with each method?

9. How would you diagnose, treat and investigate a suspected case of suxamethonium apnoea?

10. Write brief notes on the complications of blood transfusion.

11. What are the options for post-operative analgesia following a nephrectomy? State briefly the advantages and disadvantages of each.

12. What are the specific difficulties of anaesthetising an acromegalic patient for a transphenoidal hypophysectomy?

MULTIPLE CHOICE QUESTION PAPER 2

90 Questions: time allowed 3 hours.
Indicate your answers with a tick or cross in the spaces provided.

2.1 The Severinghaus electrode

❑ A consists of CO_2 sensitive glass
❑ B is better with gases than blood
❑ C is affected by nitrous oxide
❑ D contains bicarbonate ions in the electrolyte solution
❑ E measures pH

2.2 An elderly lady is dehydrated from prolonged intestinal obstruction. She is tachypnoeic and distressed, breathing air. The following are likely:

❑ A respiratory alkalosis
❑ B metabolic acidosis
❑ C hypoxaemia
❑ D uraemia
❑ E hyperglycaemia

2.3 The following are effective blocks for relieving the pain of chronic pancreatitis:

❑ A coeliac plexus
❑ B lumbar sympathetic
❑ C thoracic epidural
❑ D paravertebral
❑ E stellate ganglion

2.4 Carcinoid syndrome may be treated with

❑ A hydrocortisone
❑ B ketanserin
❑ C octreotide
❑ D Trasylol
❑ E aspirin

2.5 Soda lime

- ❑ A contains 70% calcium hydroxide and 30% sodium hydroxide
- ❑ B may not be used with sevoflurane
- ❑ C produces humidification of inspired gases
- ❑ D may warm up to 60 °C during active CO_2 absorption
- ❑ E use has been associated with carboxyhaemoglobinaemia

2.6 Sevoflurane

- ❑ A is an isomer of isoflurane
- ❑ B may cause nephrotoxicity due to its metabolism to fluoride ions
- ❑ C requires a heated vaporiser for its administration
- ❑ D is less potent than desflurane
- ❑ E causes tachycardia and hypertension at > 1 minimum alveolar concentration

2.7 Hypotension and an elevated central venous pressure may occur in

- ❑ A pulmonary embolism
- ❑ B haemorrhage
- ❑ C congestive cardiac failure
- ❑ D tension pneumothorax
- ❑ E myocardial infarction

2.8 In the management of adult VF arrest

- ❑ A the first shock should be 100 J
- ❑ B the first drug should be adrenaline 1 mg IV
- ❑ C early intravenous bicarbonate is recommended
- ❑ D bretylium tosylate is given in a dose of 5 mg/kg
- ❑ E isoprenaline is used in a dose of 5 mcg/kg

2.9 Nimodipine

❑ A is a calcium antagonist
❑ B is a cerebral protector
❑ C causes a reduced systemic vascular resistance
❑ D is contraindicated with an intravenous beta-blocker
❑ E interferes with aminophylline

2.10 Helium

❑ A has similar viscosity to oxygen
❑ B causes changes in voice
❑ C is useful treatment for bronchospasm
❑ D is stored as a liquid
❑ E supports combustion

2.11 The following occur postoperatively:

❑ A increase in nitrogen excretion
❑ B increase in K^+ excretion
❑ C increase in urinary sodium excretion
❑ D hyperglycaemia
❑ E sleep disturbances

2.12 The following suggest a difficult intubation:

❑ A Mallampatti grade 3
❑ B a thyromental distance of < 6 cm
❑ C Wilson score > 2
❑ D obesity
❑ E Parkinson's disease

2.13 Massive blood transfusion may cause

- ❑ A a coagulopathy
- ❑ B pulmonary damage
- ❑ C hypercalcaemia
- ❑ D alkalosis
- ❑ E renal failure

2.14 Acetylcholine is the neurotransmitter at

- ❑ A post-ganglionic sympathetic nerve fibres at the adrenal medulla
- ❑ B post-ganglionic sympathetic nerve fibres supplying sweat glands
- ❑ C post-ganglionic sympathetic nerve fibres supplying the bronchi
- ❑ D all autonomic ganglia
- ❑ E the neuromuscular junction

2.15 Constrictive pericarditis is associated with

- ❑ A pulsus paradoxus
- ❑ B tuberculosis
- ❑ C decreased myocardial contractility
- ❑ D pulmonary oedema
- ❑ E an elevated central venous pressure

2.16 Aortic regurgitation may occur in

- ❑ A Marfan's syndrome
- ❑ B rheumatoid arthritis
- ❑ C ankylosing spondylitis
- ❑ D syphilis
- ❑ E bacterial endocarditis

2.17 In a patient with an acute spinal cord injury

- ❑ A suxamethonium is contraindicated
- ❑ B steroids improve prognosis
- ❑ C there is usually a tachycardia
- ❑ D more than 75% of patients develop autonomic hyperreflexia
- ❑ E hypotensive anaesthesia is desirable as it reduces blood loss

2.18 The following can be used to test the integrity of the autonomic nervous system:

- ❑ A Valsalva manoeuvre
- ❑ B ephedrine
- ❑ C palpating a pulse
- ❑ D echocardiography
- ❑ E phentolamine

2.19 The incidence of deep vein thrombosis (DVT) is increased by

- ❑ A the oral contraceptive pill
- ❑ B HbSC disease
- ❑ C the lupus anticoagulant
- ❑ D polycythaemia
- ❑ E malignancy

2.20 Myxoedema coma is treated with

- ❑ A intravenous thyroxine
- ❑ B oral thyroxine
- ❑ C intravenous saline
- ❑ D intravenous hydrocortisone
- ❑ E warming the patient

2.21 Recognised features of acromegaly include

- ❑ A hypertension
- ❑ B glucose intolerance
- ❑ C dry skin
- ❑ D thyroid goitre
- ❑ E galactorrhoea

2.22 Diabetic autonomic neuropathy may result in

- ❑ A silent ischaemia
- ❑ B asystole
- ❑ C impotence
- ❑ D no pressor response to intubation
- ❑ E prolongation of the QT interval on the ECG

2.23 The bleeding time may be prolonged in

- ❑ A haemophilia A
- ❑ B von Willebrand's disease
- ❑ C disseminated intravascular coagulation (DIC)
- ❑ D vitamin K deficiency
- ❑ E scurvy

2.24 An adult patient with a prosthetic heart valve requires general anaesthesia for extraction of wisdom teeth. He should receive the following antibiotic cover:

- ❑ A gentamicin only
- ❑ B amoxycillin and gentamicin
- ❑ C vancomycin and gentamicin, if allergic to penicillin
- ❑ D no antibiotic cover
- ❑ E teicoplanin alone

2.25 The following drugs are teratogens:

❑ A lithium
❑ B warfarin
❑ C isoflurane
❑ D tetracyclines
❑ E carbamazepine

2.26 The following may be features of the TUR syndrome:

❑ A hypotension with bradycardia
❑ B confusion
❑ C hypernatraemia
❑ D haemolysis
❑ E disseminated intravascular coagulation

2.27 Ropivacaine

❑ A has an identical pKa to bupivacaine
❑ B is less cardiotoxic than bupivacaine
❑ C is more potent than bupivacaine
❑ D produces greater motor block than bupivacaine
❑ E is a pure enantiomer

2.28 Fat embolism can cause

❑ A a petechial rash
❑ B central cyanosis
❑ C pyrexia
❑ D cerebral oedema
❑ E carbon dioxide retention

2.29 The recurrent laryngeal nerve

- ❑ A supplies the sensory fibres to the larynx below the vocal cords
- ❑ B supplies the motor fibres to some intrinsic muscles of the larynx
- ❑ C crosses the inferior thyroid artery or its branches
- ❑ D supplies the motor fibres to the cricothyroid muscle
- ❑ E supplies the inferior constrictor muscle of the pharynx

2.30 The following may cause convulsions:

- ❑ A hypomagnesaemia
- ❑ B hypercalcaemia
- ❑ C enflurane
- ❑ D hyponatraemia
- ❑ E anaemia

2.31 The following are found in hyperparathyroidism:

- ❑ A extraosseous calcification
- ❑ B renal calculi
- ❑ C raised plasma calcium
- ❑ D lowered urinary calcium
- ❑ E increased urinary phosphate

2.32 Lower oesophageal tone is increased by

- ❑ A metoclopramide
- ❑ B atropine
- ❑ C domperidone
- ❑ D morphine
- ❑ E cisapride

2.33 Magnesium

- ❑ A is the anticonvulsant of choice in eclampsia
- ❑ B readily crosses the placenta
- ❑ C potentiates the action of non-depolarising muscle relaxants
- ❑ D overdosage causes cardiac arrest
- ❑ E deficiency causes prolongation of the QT interval on the ECG

2.34 Alfentanil

- ❑ A is less lipid-soluble than fentanyl
- ❑ B is more potent than fentanyl
- ❑ C has a longer half-life than fentanyl
- ❑ D is shorter acting than fentanyl
- ❑ E has several active metabolites

2.35 Radial nerve palsy causes

- ❑ A inability to extend the elbow
- ❑ B inability to extend the wrist
- ❑ C inability to pronate the forearm
- ❑ D loss of sensation at the base of the thumb
- ❑ E wasting of the thenar eminence

2.36 Papilloedema can

- ❑ A be caused by central retinal artery occlusion
- ❑ B be caused by central retinal vein occlusion
- ❑ C be caused by cavernous sinus thrombosis
- ❑ D be unilateral
- ❑ E occur with pulmonary oedema

2.37 Non-steroidal anti-inflammatory drugs

- ❑ A are useful postoperative analgesics
- ❑ B may cause thrombocytopenia
- ❑ C can be given intrathecally
- ❑ D inhibit cyclo-oxygenase
- ❑ E can precipitate renal failure

2.38 The following would alert you to the need to increase respiratory support:

- ❑ A tired and sweating
- ❑ B mouth open and tracheal tug
- ❑ C use of platysma
- ❑ D flaring of the ala nasae
- ❑ E bounding peripheral pulses

2.39 The following are essential criteria for brain stem death:

- ❑ A equal pupils
- ❑ B absent limb movements
- ❑ C doll's eye movements
- ❑ D $paCO_2$ > 6.7 kPa at the end of apnoea
- ❑ E normal blood glucose

2.40 The pulse oximeter may be inaccurate if

- ❑ A there is carboxyhaemoglobin present
- ❑ B there is marked vasoconstriction
- ❑ C the patient is dark skinned
- ❑ D there is a high concentration of HbF
- ❑ E there is tricuspid regurgitation

2.41 The following may cause a metabolic alkalosis:

- ❑ A Cushing's syndrome
- ❑ B gastrocolic fistula
- ❑ C acetazolamide
- ❑ D pyloric stenosis
- ❑ E carbenoxolone therapy

2.42 Trigeminal neuralgia

- ❑ A affects the sixth cranial nerve
- ❑ B when the ophthalmic branch of the trigeminal nerve is affected there is loss of the corneal reflex
- ❑ C is successfully treated with carbamazepine
- ❑ D may be intractable
- ❑ E may be the presenting feature in multiple sclerosis

2.43 An arterial line in the radial artery can lead to

- ❑ A fatal haemorrhage
- ❑ B pulmonary embolism
- ❑ C intracerebral embolism
- ❑ D parasthaesia at the base of the thumb
- ❑ E septicaemia

2.44 In an exponential process

- ❑ A time constant and half-life are synonymous
- ❑ B 37% of the process is completed in one time constant
- ❑ C 95% of the process is completed in three time constants
- ❑ D rate of change is constant
- ❑ E washout curves are exponential processes

2.45 In an unconscious patient the following clinical signs suggest a cervical cord injury:

- ❑ A hypotension with bradycardia
- ❑ B diaphragmatic breathing
- ❑ C priapism
- ❑ D flaccid areflexia of the limbs
- ❑ E a fixed, dilated pupil

2.46 Etomidate

- ❑ A is an imidazole
- ❑ B has an ester link
- ❑ C causes greater post-operative nausea and vomiting than propofol
- ❑ D has a low incidence of allergy
- ❑ E is contraindicated in porphyria

2.47 Regarding malignant hyperpyrexia

- ❑ A it is associated with central core disease
- ❑ B it may be precipitated by isoflurane
- ❑ C dantrolene is the specific treatment
- ❑ D it is inherited as an autosomal recessive gene
- ❑ E the local anaesthetic agents are safe

2.48 Treatment of air embolism during posterior cranial fossa surgery includes

- ❑ A increasing intracranial venous pressure
- ❑ B rapid intravenous fluids
- ❑ C mannitol
- ❑ D placing the patient laterally, right side down
- ❑ E increasing the nitrous oxide

2.49 Amniotic fluid embolism

- ❑ A can occur more than 24 hours after delivery
- ❑ B can occur after a therapeutic abortion
- ❑ C can only be diagnosed definitely at post mortem
- ❑ D is commoner if a syntocinon infusion is used
- ❑ E there is often an associated coagulopathy

2.50 Crystalloid cardioplegic solutions

- ❑ A contain high concentrations of calcium
- ❑ B contain high concentrations of potassium
- ❑ C contain procaine
- ❑ D stop the heart in diastole
- ❑ E may contain magnesium

2.51 Concerning an ankle block

- ❑ A there are four nerves to be blocked
- ❑ B apart from the saphenous nerve, all the other nerves to be blocked are derived from the sciatic nerve
- ❑ C the sural nerve lies anterior to the lateral malleolus
- ❑ D the tibial nerve lies deep to the posterior tibial artery
- ❑ E the deep peroneal nerve lies lateral to the anterior tibial artery

2.52 Disseminated intravascular coagulation (DIC) may occur in

- ❑ A amniotic fluid embolus
- ❑ B acute promyelocytic leukaemia
- ❑ C falciparum malaria
- ❑ D haemolytic transfusion reaction.
- ❑ E thrombotic thrombocytopenic purpura

2.53 In acute liver failure

- ❑ A a prothrombin time > 20 seconds indicates severe failure
- ❑ B the level of serum alanine aminotransferase (LDH) is a sensitive marker
- ❑ C the serum bilirubin is a sensitive marker
- ❑ D paracetamol may be implicated aetiologically
- ❑ E halothane may be implicated aetiologically

2.54 The following may be complications of tracheostomy:

- ❑ A pneumothorax
- ❑ B tracheal stenosis
- ❑ C haemorrhage
- ❑ D surgical emphysema
- ❑ E cardiovascular collapse

2.55 Blood cell antigen A

- ❑ A has Mendelian inheritance
- ❑ B is less common than B
- ❑ C is the main cause of haemolytic disease of the newborn
- ❑ D is found in all RBCs
- ❑ E is found in saliva

2.56 Left ventricular failure is a more likely diagnosis than asthma in the presence of

- ❑ A early cyanosis
- ❑ B a raised jugular venous pressure (JVP)
- ❑ C expiratory rhonchi
- ❑ D inspiratory basal crepitations
- ❑ E shadowing on the chest X-ray (CXR)

2.57 The following values are less in obstructive than in restrictive lung disease:

- ❑ A functional residual capacity (FRC)
- ❑ B FEV1 / FVC
- ❑ C peak expiratory flow rate (PEFR)
- ❑ D carbon monoxide transfer factor (TLCO)
- ❑ E tidal volume (TV)

2.58 Erythropoietin production

- ❑ A is reduced in renal disease
- ❑ B is stimulated by hypercarbia
- ❑ C is increased in chronic obstructive airways disease
- ❑ D is reduced at altitude
- ❑ E takes place in the bone marrow

2.59 Concerning the oxyhaemoglobin dissociation curve

- ❑ A the P75 is 5.3 kPa
- ❑ B it is shifted to the right in chronic anaemia
- ❑ C it is shifted to the left in hypoventilation
- ❑ D it is unaffected by temperature
- ❑ E it is shifted to the right in carbon monoxide poisoning

2.60 The following are associated with rheumatoid arthritis:

- ❑ A pericardial effusion
- ❑ B haemolytic anaemia
- ❑ C constrictive pericarditis
- ❑ D renal failure
- ❑ E tricuspid incompetence

2.61 Concerning the neonatal airway

- ❑ A the trachea is 4 cm long
- ❑ B the larynx is at C5
- ❑ C the epiglottis is U-shaped
- ❑ D the tracheal rings are not fully formed
- ❑ E the cricoid is the narrowest part of the airway

2.62 Fallot's tetralogy is associated with

- ❑ A squatting
- ❑ B syncope
- ❑ C murmur due to continuous flow through a VSD
- ❑ D overriding pulmonary artery
- ❑ E aortic stenosis

2.63 Hypofibrinogenaemia occurs with

- ❑ A DIC
- ❑ B the oral contraceptive pill
- ❑ C asparaginase
- ❑ D prostate resection
- ❑ E massive transfusion

2.64 Morphine

- ❑ A may cause inappropriate ADH release
- ❑ B is metabolised to morphine-6-glucuronide
- ❑ C is an antiemetic
- ❑ D stimulates the Edinger-Westphal nucleus
- ❑ E stimulates the chemoreceptor trigger zone

2.65 Retrobulbar block

- ❑ A prevents lacrimation
- ❑ B causes papilloedema
- ❑ C causes enophthalmos
- ❑ D decreases intraocular pressure
- ❑ E causes miosis

2.66 Concerning phaeochromocytomata

- ❑ A 10% are familial
- ❑ B they may cause hypotension
- ❑ C they may cause hypertension
- ❑ D they may secrete adrenaline, noradrenaline or dopamine
- ❑ E they are a cause of secondary diabetes insipidus

2.67 Myaesthenia gravis

- ❑ A only occurs in females
- ❑ B is associated with anti-acetylcholine receptor antibodies
- ❑ C patients are resistant to non-depolarising muscle relaxants
- ❑ D may be treated by plasmaphaeresis
- ❑ E is often due to an underlying oat cell carcinoma of the bronchus

2.68 Mitral stenosis is associated with

- ❑ A a loud first heart sound
- ❑ B an early diastolic murmur
- ❑ C a displaced apex beat
- ❑ D a malar flush
- ❑ E atrial fibrillation

2.69 Two days post abdominal surgery the following observations are recorded: blood pressure 80/40, pulse 100/min, temperature 39 °C central venous pressure 2 cm H_2O. This could be due to

- ❑ A myocardial infarct
- ❑ B septicaemia
- ❑ C basal atelectasis
- ❑ D anastomotic breakdown
- ❑ E cardiac tamponade

2.70 Coronary artery blood flow

- ❑ A occurs mainly in diastole
- ❑ B is autoregulated
- ❑ C is reduced by tachycardia
- ❑ D accounts for about 5% of the cardiac output
- ❑ E is reduced if the venous pressure falls

2.71 An increased tidal volume is a recognised manifestation of

- ❑ A ankylosing spondylitis
- ❑ B diabetic ketoacidosis
- ❑ C emphysema
- ❑ D cerebral haemorrhage
- ❑ E uraemia

2.72 The specific gravity of urine is reduced in

- ❑ A diabetes insipidus
- ❑ B acute tubular necrosis
- ❑ C intestinal obstruction
- ❑ D lithium toxicity
- ❑ E diabetes mellitus

2.73 The hazard of microshock in hospital can be reduced by the use of

- ❑ A isolated (floating) power supply
- ❑ B saline-filled intracardiac catheters
- ❑ C battery powered appliances
- ❑ D multiple earth paths
- ❑ E large area diathermy plate

2.74 The following drugs cross the blood-brain barrier:

- ❑ A L-Dopa
- ❑ B atropine
- ❑ C neostigmine
- ❑ D mannitol
- ❑ E fentanyl

2.75 The speed of uptake of an anaesthetic agent from the lung

- ❑ A is proportional to the cardiac output
- ❑ B is proportional to the minute ventilation
- ❑ C is proportional to the minimum alveolar concentration
- ❑ D is proportional to the blood gas solubility
- ❑ E is temperature dependent

2.76 Diabetic amyotrophy

- ❑ A affects predominantly the distal muscles of the lower limbs
- ❑ B is associated with an increase in cerebrospinal fluid protein
- ❑ C usually responds to improved blood sugar control
- ❑ D causes impotence
- ❑ E causes urinary retention

2.77 A patient who has vomited, presents with acute abdominal pain. On examination he is noted to have epigastric guarding, laboured respiration, slight cyanosis and subcutaneous emphysema in the neck. This suggests

- ❑ A pulmonary infarction
- ❑ B ruptured diaphragm
- ❑ C spontaneous pneumothorax
- ❑ D ruptured oesophagus
- ❑ E ruptured trachea

2.78 Dystrophia myotonica is associated with

- ❑ A sterility
- ❑ B dysarthria
- ❑ C cataracts
- ❑ D temporalis muscle wasting
- ❑ E sternomastoid muscle wasting

2.79 The following clinical findings occur in the Brown-Sequard syndrome:

- ❑ A contralateral weakness
- ❑ B ipsilateral extensor plantar responses
- ❑ C contralateral loss of pain and temperature sensation
- ❑ D ipsilateral loss of awareness of vibration
- ❑ E Rombergism

2.80 Vomiting may be associated with

- ❑ A metabolic alkalosis
- ❑ B alkaline urine
- ❑ C raised plasma chloride levels
- ❑ D hyperkalaemia
- ❑ E elevated blood urea

2.81 The complications of Crohn's disease include

- ❑ A entero-enteric fistula formation
- ❑ B recurrence following excision of the primary lesion
- ❑ C fistula in ano
- ❑ D lymphoma
- ❑ E polyarthritis

2.82 Recognised causes of glycosuria include

- ❑ A phaeochromocytoma
- ❑ B pregnancy
- ❑ C partial gastrectomy
- ❑ D hypopituitarism
- ❑ E subarachnoid haemorrhage

2.83 Cardiac tamponade

- ❑ A may complicate aortic dissection
- ❑ B produces a rise in jugular venous pressure
- ❑ C causes a small radial pulse which fades on inspiration
- ❑ D is different from congestive cardiac failure (CCF) in not causing hepatomegaly
- ❑ E is best treated by a vigorous diuretic regime

2.84 In electrocardiography

- ❑ A a potassium ion gradient is mainly responsible for the electrical potential difference across the cell membrane
- ❑ B an exploring electrode records an upward deflection when the depolarisation current is flowing away from it
- ❑ C the PR interval is reduced in first degree heart block
- ❑ D the QT interval is reduced in hypocalcaemia
- ❑ E the T wave is due to ventricular repolarisation

2.85 Ketamine

- ❑ A has minimal analgesic properties
- ❑ B may provoke bronchospasm
- ❑ C is an antagonist at the NMDA receptor
- ❑ D is presented as a racemic mixture
- ❑ E is an appropriate agent for the induction of patients with haemorrhagic shock

2.86 Complications of long-term spironolactone therapy include

- ❑ A metabolic alkalosis
- ❑ B hyponatraemia
- ❑ C hypoglycaemia
- ❑ D hyperkalaemia
- ❑ E hyperuricaemia

2.87 Propranolol administered intravenously

- ❑ A decreases airway resistance
- ❑ B causes hyperglycaemia
- ❑ C decreases the inotropic action of digitalis
- ❑ D is dangerous in patients receiving verapamil
- ❑ E is the agent of chioce for the treatment of ventricular ectopic beats in a patient with an acute myocardial infarct

2.88 The following are commonly seen with acute salicylate poisoning:

- ❑ A fibrinolysis
- ❑ B respiratory acidosis
- ❑ C high output renal failure
- ❑ D hypothermia
- ❑ E massive gastric bleeding

2.89 In patients with untreated megaloblastic anaemia

- ❑ A histamine fast achlorhydria is always present
- ❑ B there may be a peripheral neuropathy
- ❑ C there is an increased incidence of carcinoma of the stomach
- ❑ D resection of the ileum for Crohn's disease may be causally related
- ❑ E the serum B12 level may be within the normal range

2.90 Estimation of prothrombin time is useful in

- ❑ A haemophilia
- ❑ B von Willebrand's disease
- ❑ C scurvy
- ❑ D jaundice
- ❑ E thrombocytopenic purpura

PRACTICE EXAM 2: THE CLINICAL VIVAS

Viva 1: The Clinical Viva takes place in the morning.

1. You are given a piece of clinical information and you have 10 minutes to study it.
2. You will spend 20 minutes with the first examiner, discussing the clinical care of the patient described and how you would anaesthetise for the case.
3. You will then spend 20 minutes with a second examiner discussing approximately three unrelated clinical scenarios.

Viva 2: The Clinical Science Viva takes place in the afternoon. Two examiners will question you for approximately 15 minutes each. Approximately four topics are covered.

A good way to prepare for the viva is to work with a partner. For this reason we have separated the sample questions in this book from the model answers to allow you to work through the viva session before looking at the answers.

Viva 1

Clinical Scenario

A previously fit and well 26 year-old primigravida at 32/40 weeks' gestation complains of increasingly painful paraesthesia of the thumb and index finger of her left hand.

Examination reveals pulse 100 beats/minutes, blood pressure 110/70. There are first and second heart sounds plus a systolic murmur best heard in the aortic area. There is oedema of the legs bilaterally.

Laboratory investigations:

Hb	9.9 g/dl	WCC	11.9 x 10^9/l	Pts	156 x 10^9/l

Haemoglobin electrophoresis: HbA and HbS detected

Na	130 mmol/l	K	4.2 mmol/l	Urea	2.1 mmol/l

Albumin 29 g/l
ALP 356 (norm. 60-110)
24 hr urinary protein 150mg
PT 12 secs

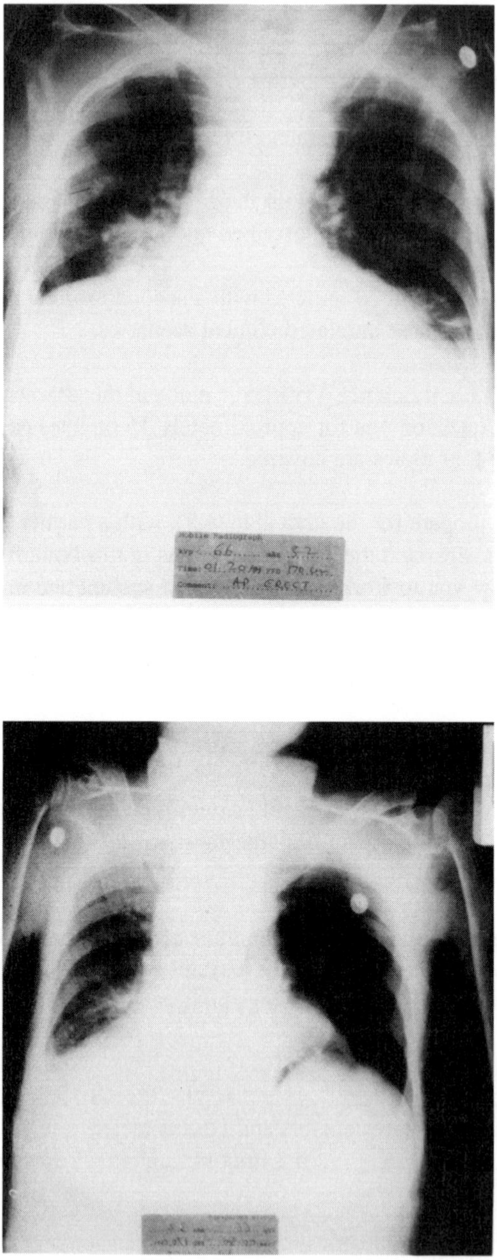

Fig. 3: Chest X-rays

Examiner 1

Summarise this case.

What is carpal tunnel syndrome?

Comment on the physical findings and laboratory investigations.

How would you anaesthetise this patient?

Examiner 2

What does this CXR show? (Fig. 3) Shortly after this CXR was taken the lady developed severe respiratory distress, cyanosis and a barely palpable pulse.
What is your management?

Tell me about eye blocks for cataract surgery.

Tell me about the problems associated with acute "ecstasy" intoxication.

Viva 2

Examiner 1

Tell me about inotropes.

Tell me about the problems of anaesthesia at high altitude.

Examiner 2

Tell me about postoperative nausea and vomiting.

Tell me about the predication of difficult intubation.

SHORT ANSWER QUESTION PAPER 2 ANSWERS

1. ***How would you pre-operatively assess, investigate and resuscitate a 6-week-old infant prior to repair of congenital hypertrophic pyloric stenosis?***

- Usually males, often low birth weight presenting with projectile vomiting following feeds (though constantly hungry) at 2–6 weeks of age. Approximately 1 in 350 live births.

- Vomiting produces dehydration and metabolic imbalance. Dehydration assessed clinically:
  a) 5% loss, mild, dry mucous membranes.
  b) 10% loss, moderate, mottled cold peripheries, poor capillary refill, sunken fontanelle, oliguria and hypotension.
  c) 15% loss, severe, shocked and moribund.

- Metabolic imbalance, loss of gastric hydrogen and chloride ions produces hypochloraemic alkalosis. Initially, the kidney conserves hydrogen ions in exchange for potassium but, with severe dehydration, sodium retention predominates in exchange for hydrogen producing an acid urine. The end result is a hypochloraemic, hypokalaemic metabolic alkalosis with compensatory hypoventilation.

- Pre-operative resuscitation is essential. Surgery is not an emergency.
  a) Nasogastric tube passed, aspirated frequently, nil by mouth instituted. Blood sugar should be monitored as hypoglycaemia may occur.
  b) Intravenous fluid replacement. 0.9% Saline with potassium supplements: Initially 50 ml/kg; 100 ml/kg or 150 ml/kg according to mild-severe dehydration and repeated according to response, electrolyte measurements and urine output.
  c) Confirmation of resuscitation prior to surgery:
     Serum sodium > 135 mmol/l
     Serum chloride > 90 mmol/l
     Serum bicarbonate < 30mmol/l.

Ref: BJA 1987: 59; 672–677.

2. *What are the preconditions for testing and how would you perform brain stem death testing?*

The preconditions for testing are:
- Apnoeic coma requiring ventilation
- Known cause of irreversible brain damage – usually confirmed by CT head scan.

Patients must be excluded if:
- Hypothermic (core temp < 35 °C)
- Central depressant or muscle relaxant drugs are present
- No severe acid/base abnormality or severe metabolic disease (e.g. profound hyponatraemia, uraemia hepatic encephalopathy)
- Uncontrolled endocrine disease (e.g. hypothyroidism or diabetes mellitus)
- Markedly elevated $PaCO_2$
- Severe hypotension.

Brain stem function tests:
1. Pupillary reflexes – no direct or consensual reaction to light. Tests CNII and PNS
2. Corneal reflexes – no response to light touching cornea tests CNV and CNIII
3. Oculocephalic reflexes remain in fixed position within orbit when head is rotated from side to side. Test CN VIII
4. Caloric tests – after visualizing the tympanic membranes both sides, 30 ml ice cold water is injected into external auditory meatus. No nystagmus is seen if there is no brain stem function. Tests CN VIII
5. No response to painful stimulus applied to the face (usually pressure to the supra orbital fissure) Tests CN V and VIL
6. Gag reflex absent during stimulation of oropharynx. Tests IX and X
7. Apnoea test – following ventilation with 100% O_2 patient is disconnected from ventilator (continuing passive insufflation of 6 l O_2/min) There is no respiratory effort during this time despite drive from a rising $PaCO_2$. An ABG is taken to prove the $PaCO_2$ is above 7.6 kPa.

3. ***A primigravid woman is found collapsed in the delivery suite following an epidural 'top-up' administered by the midwife 5 minutes before. List the likely causes and the initial management.***

Causes:
- Aorto caval compression, impaired venous return causing low cardiac output.
- Intravascular administration of local anaesthetic, central nervous system toxicity causing convulsions followed by cardiovascular collapse.
- Subarachnoid administration of local anaesthetic causing total spinal.
- Other causes to which the temporal relationship to the 'top-up' was circumstantial (e.g. massive antepartum haemorrhage or amniotic fluid embolus).

Initial management:
- Call for senior help: senior anaesthetist, obstetrician and midwife
- Turn the patient onto the left lateral position or wedge to relieve any aorto caval compression.
- Assess the airway and breathing, control the airway if necessary by intubation and administer high flow oxygen by face mask or IPPV.
- Assess the circulation, gain intravenous access with at least one 14G cannula and monitor the ECG.
- Give intravenous fluids and vasopressors or inotropes to improve the circulation. If there is no cardiac output follow the advanced life support algorithms remembering that ventricular fibrillation following intravenous bupivacaine is resistant to conventional therapy and may require bretylium.
- Send samples for crossmatch and send for emergency O-negative blood if uncontrolled haemorrhage is present.
- Frequently assess both the maternal and fetal response to therapy.
- Early discussion with the obstetrician of the mode of fetal delivery.

4. ***A previously fit 30-year-old male sustains an isolated fracture of the femur during a motor cycle accident. Six hours after admission he becomes dyspnoeic. What are the likely causes and their initial management?***

Possible causes:
- simple pneumothorax
- tension pneumothorax
- haemothorax
- fat embolism
- occult haemorrhage causing hypovolaemia.

Management:
- Give supplemental oxygen while obtaining diagnostic chest X-ray and arterial blood gas analysis, if the clinical situation allows.
- Assess the circulation and obtain intravenous access with large bore cannula. Give fluid as appropriate.
- Simple pneumothorax will require percutaneous thoracostomy tube for decompression while a tension pneumothorax (with cardiovascular compromise and a markedly deviated trachea) will require emergency decompression with a 14 G cannula prior to thoracostomy tube.
- Haemothorax will require drainage via a thoracostomy tube; though this may cause worsened haemodynamic instability once the tamponading effect of the blood is removed.
- Sources of occult haemorrhage such as intra-abdominal should be sought, these may require surgical intervention.
- Fat embolism syndrome will present with hypoxaemia and hypocarbia due to shunting of blood in the lungs which are obstructed by micro fat emboli.
- Chest X-ray may be normal, there may be a petechial rash over the trunk and conjunctivae, fat droplets may be found in sputum and urine.

Management is supportive; maintenance of oxygenation with supplemental oxygen or intermittent positive pressure ventilation. Early fixation of long bone fractures may reduce ongoing embolization.

5. ***Describe your management of an adult patient brought into the accident and emergency department in status epilepticus.***

Definition: A seizure or series of seizures lasting longer than 30 minutes without regaining consciousness. Mortality 2.5% and morbidity including focal neurological deficits, intellectual deterioration and chronic epilepsy make it a medical emergency.

Management comprises control of convulsion and investigation of aetiology. Initial management:

- Maintain airway, give high flow oxygen via face mask, monitor vital signs – ECG, pulse oximetry and blood pressure.
- Gain intravenous access, give intravenous diazepam in 5 mg doses up to 20 mg.
- Obtain blood for analysis of blood count, electrolytes (including Ca), blood glucose, serum anti-convulsant levels and toxicology screen.
- Give phenytoin 15 mg/kg as slow intravenous infusion with close monitoring (may cause hypotension and dysrhythmias).
- If seizures persist second-line therapy should take place on the intensive therapy unit as drugs used may cause hypoventilation, loss of airway reflexes and intubation may be required. Second-line therapy of thiopentone infusion 3–5 mg/kg bolus followed by 1–3 mg/kg/hr with cardiorespiratory support.
- If continuing tonic clonic convulsions compromise oxygenation neuromuscular paralysis may be considered with continuous EEG monitoring to detect further convulsions.
- Investigation into aetiology: 25% of patients have idiopathic epilepsy; drug non-compliance causing status. 75% of patients have either a brain lesion or metabolic derangement, commonly alcohol withdrawal, cerebrovascular lesion, drug intoxication (e.g. theophylline or tricyclics) or a space occupying brain lesion.
- Differentiation will include both biochemical investigation and imaging via CT or MRI.

Ref: Anaesthesia 1995: 50; 130–135.

6. ***How may nutrition be provided for patients on the intensive care unit? What are the advantages and disadvantages of each?***

Enteral feeding:
Provided via fine bore nasogastric or enterostomy tube. Ideal feed is osmolar delivered in a controlled manner to prevent gastric distension. Providing 1.5 g/kg/day protein and 32–40 kcal/kg/day as well as vitamins and minerals. Preferable since cheap, physiological, protects gut from erosions via physical barrier and increasing splanchnic blood flow. Recent evidence suggests reduction in villous atrophy, incidence of nosocomial pneumonia and translocation of toxins across the gut wall. Requires an intact functioning gut (> 25 cm of ileum needed). May be contraindicated with intra-abdominal pathologies (e.g. pancreatitis, post surgical bowel resection). Complications include: misplaced tube, gastric distension and aspiration, diarrhoea, bacterial contamination of feed, variable absorption.

Parenteral feeding:
Used in the absence of functioning gut. Provided as a hyperosmolar solution, administered into a central vein. Protein requirement assessed by monitoring daily urinary urea production, each gram of nitrogen matched by 100–125 kcals of energy. Variable absorption is not a problem. Complications are numerous and frequent. Central venous cannulation has significant complications, sepsis of the line site and septicaemia in up to 25% of patients. Metabolic derangements: hyperglycaemia, electrolyte imbalance (K, Mg, Ph), hyperlipoproteinaemia, hypercholesterolaemia, fatty infiltration of the liver.

7. ***What are the indications for intubation in the adult? How may the airway be anaesthetised prior to intubation?***

Indications:

- Anatomically deformed upper airway, especially if anaesthesia may lead to loss of that airway.
- Inability to open mouth.
- To avoid aspiration in patients with a full stomach.
- Respiratory failure requiring ventilation, to avoid the cardiac depressant effects of anaesthetic drugs.

Airway anaesthesia may be provided by several means:

- Lignocaine nebulizer, 3 ml 4% lignocaine over 10–20 minutes.
- Cocaine solution 4% (2.5 ml for 70 kg person) to the nasal mucosa. Superior laryngeal nerve block with a 23 G needle 3 ml 1% lignocaine is injected near the inferior border of the greater cornu of the hyoid bone bilaterally. Recurrent laryngeal nerve block by trans-tracheal injection of 3–5 ml of 1% lignocaine using a 23 G needle via the cricothyroid membrane. The oropharynx either by sucking an amethocaine lozenge or by direct spray.
- Cocaine solution as before provides anaesthesia of the nasal mucosa. The fibre optic intubating scope is inserted and small amounts of 4% lignocaine are injected as it is advanced.

8. ***How may gas exchange and anaesthesia be maintained during rigid bronchoscopy? What problems are associated with each method?***

Deep anaesthesia with spontaneous respiration.
Classically children. Anaesthetic gases (usually nitrous oxide, oxygen, halothane mixture) are delivered via the side arm of the ventilating bronchoscope. Deep anaesthesia is required to tolerate instrumentation and may lead to toxicity from halothane. High resistance to breathing. Anaesthesia will lighten when the eye piece is removed for biopsy/retrieval of foreign bodies.

Paralysis and controlled ventilation with light anaesthesia.
Methods of maintaining gas exchange during paralysis:

- Apnoeic insufflation: suitable for short procedures as $PaCO_2$ rises 0.4 kPa/min. Intermittent ventilation to control the rise.
- Ventilating bronchoscope. Children especially may be hand ventilated using an Ayres T piece attached to the side arm of the bronchoscope. Changes in compliance or airway obstruction detected easily but no ventilation when the eye piece is opened.
- Sanders injector. Injection of 4 Bar oxygen via 16 G injection port. Obstruction to outflow will cause barotrauma, unsuitable for young children. Entrainment of variable amounts of air causing unknown FiO_2.
- High frequency positive pressure ventilation. Enables lower mean airway pressures with no air entrainment. High flow out of the bronchoscope risks debris being carried towards the operator. Maintenance of anaesthesia in these cases tends to be via intermittent boluses of relaxant together with continuous infusion of intravenous anaesthetic agent.

9. ***How would you diagnose, treat and investigate a suspected case of suxamethonium apnoea?***

Prolonged paralysis may be caused by:

- Reduced cholinesterase activity due to inherited atypical cholinesterase, reduced amount of cholinesterase (e.g. severe chronic liver disease or pregnancy) or inhibition of cholinesterase by drugs (e.g. ecothiopate).
- Excessive dosage; cumulation of suxamethonium and production of a dual block.

Management:

- Maintenance of anaesthesia and oxygenation.
- Diagnosis of the nature of the block using neuromuscular blockade monitoring. With dual block there will be fade during the train of four and edrophonium will improve the fade whereas with prolonged depolarizing blockade there is no fade (or more usually no response at all).
- Neostigmine has been used to reverse dual blockade.
- Spontaneous recovery, usually within 4 hours occurs with prolonged depolarizing blockade. This may be speeded by the administration of blood or plasma but spontaneous recovery is preferable.
- Following recovery, blood may be analysed for cholinesterase activity by the degree of enzyme inhibition by dibucaine or fluoride. (Normal dibucaine No 75–85, fluoride No 60.)
- Atypical enzyme (0.03% population are homozygotes) dibucaine No 15-25 and fluoride No 20. Silent gene (0.001% population are homozygotes). No plasma cholinesterase activity. Fluoride resistant gene (0.0001% population are homozygotes).
- Full explanation to the patient should be given with consideration of a 'medi-alert' bracelet and screening of other family members.

10. Write brief notes on the complications of blood transfusion.

May be classified into early and late.

Early immunological:
- Haemolytic immediate (ABO) incompatibility
- IgM cold antibodies
- In the awake patient dyspnoea, chest pain and loin pain precede cardiovascular collapse
- In the anaesthetised patient hypotension, fever, and DIC occur
- Reaction to leucocytes, platelets and plasma proteins causing fever and hypotension
- Graft versus host disease in immunocompromised patients
- Transfusion of infected blood. Septicaemia from Gram-negative organisms (rare)
- Circulatory overload
- Air embolism, thrombophlebitis
- Metabolic: hyperkalaemia (rarely a problem) potassium is taken up into cells as they rewarm, hypocalcaemia due to citrate toxicity only in massive transfusion, acid/base disturbance
- Coagulopathy: dilution of platelets and lack of factors.

Late immunological:
- Rh incompatibility IgG antibodies cause jaundice and haemolytic anaemia 7–8 days following transfusion
- May cause haemolytic disease of the newborn in rhesus-negative mothers
- Transmission of infection
- Viral: Hepatitis B or C, HIV, CMV
- Bacterial: *Treponema, Brucella, Salmonella*
- Parasites: malaria, *Toxoplasma*
- Iron overload.

11. What are the options for post-operative analgesia following a nephrectomy? State briefly the advantages and disadvantages of each.

Options broadly divided into systemic or regional.

Systemic:

- Intermittent intramuscular opiate: technically easy, high safety profile, either on prn basis or regular administration. Involves difficulties with nursing delays, patients reluctance to ask for analgaesia, peaks and troughs in plasma opiate concentrations with periods of inadequate pain control.
- Patient controlled analgesia systems: involves use of high tech pumps allowing the patient to control the amount of opiate required according to the level of pain. Patient must be able to understand and be physically able to operate the button. Side-effects of respiratory depression, nausea, vomiting and pruritis may be a problem.
- Systemic paracetamol may be used as an adjunct though non-steroidals are generally avoided acutely due to potential renal toxicity.

Regional:

- Intercostal nerve blockade: usually performed at the time of surgery, during surgical exposure of the neurovascular bundle. Last a fixed period of time following surgery. A catheter may be left *in situ* for repeated boluses however multiple blocks are necessary for full analgaesia.
- Epidural analgesia: technically more difficult and invasive with complications (dural puncture, infection, hypotension) and requiring high level of monitoring to avoid potentially serious side-effects. Block may be ineffective or cause disturbing motor paralysis of the lower limbs.

12. *What are the specific difficulties of anaesthetising an acromegalic patient for a transphenoidal hypophysectomy?*

Acromegalic patients pose a number of difficult problems:

- Tissue hypertrophy with an enlarged tongue and soft tissues will predispose to airway difficulties.
- Up to 50% of patients have obstructive sleep apnoea and may lose their airway on induction of anaesthesia.
- Co-existing disease is common; hypertension, left ventricular hypertrophy or failure and coronary artery disease occur frequently. Impaired glucose tolerance and diabetes mellitus occur in 25% of patients.
- Premedication. Continuation of regular medication, especially anti-hypertensives, may require insulin, avoid sedative medication if sleep apnoea, an anti-sialagogue may be helpful if a difficult intubation is anticipated.
- Intubation may require use of a fibre optic intubating scope. A flexo-metallic endotracheal tube is inserted to avoid kinking. A throat pack and preparation of the nasal mucosa using cocaine paste.
- Major haemorrhage may occur peri-operatively as the carotid artery traverses the carotid sinus near to the surgical field.
- Post-operative nursing on an high dependency unit with frequent neurological observations, close monitoring of blood glucose and urine output. Diabetes insipidus is common and may require treatment with DDAVP.

Ref: Current Anaesthesia & Critical Care 1993: 4; 8–12.

MCQ PAPER 2 ANSWERS

2.1 Severinghaus electrode **Answers: D E**

The in vitro carbon dioxide electrode (Severinghaus) is used to measure the tension of carbon dioxide in blood; $PaCO_2$. The pH is what is actually measured; this is directly related to $PaCO_2$ since:
$CO_2 + H_2O \rightarrow H_2CO_3 \rightarrow H^+ + HCO_3^-$. CO_2 in the blood diffuses across a semimpermeable membrane. The above reaction then occurs at the pH sensitive glass electrode, which is bathed in bicarbonate solution. The pH is measured from which the $PaCO_2$ is then calculated.

2.2 Prolonged intestinal obstruction **Answers: A B C D**

Prolonged intestinal obstruction leads to dehydration and uraemia. The patient usually develops a metabolic acidosis and a compensatory respiratory alkalosis. The patient might well be hypoxic if only breathing room air, but there is no particular reason for hyperglycaemia.

2.3 Chronic pancreatitis **Answers: A C**

Coeliac plexus block is the one most often used to treat the pain of chronic pancreatitis. It may also be used to treat the pain of pancreatic cancer. A stellate ganglion block is used to block the sympathetic innervation of the face and arm.

2.4 Carcinoid syndrome **Answers: B C D**

The carcinoid syndrome is due to the effects of serotonin, which is produced by a tumour, usually in the ileum. The syndrome only occurs in the presence of hepatic secondaries. It may lead to intermittent wheezing, diarrhoea and flushing as well as right-sided cardiac valvular lesions such as tricuspid stenosis. Medical treatment includes octreotide, ketanserin and cyproheptadine. Aprotinin (Trasylol) may also be used, as it prevents the peripheral conversion of kallikrein to bradykinin, which some tumours secrete.

2.5 Soda lime **Answers: C D E**

Soda lime is used to absorb CO_2 in anaesthetic breathing systems. It contains approximately 90% calcium hydroxide. Sodium hydroxide (5%) and potassium hydroxide (1%) are present as catalysts for the reaction between soda lime and CO_2. An indicator dye is present to show when the soda lime is exhausted. In the most often used soda lime (Durasorb) the dye is Clayton yellow, which turns from pink to yellow.

The reaction is:
$2NaOH + CO_2 \rightarrow Na_2CO_3 + H_2O$ and then:
$Na_2CO_3 + Ca(OH)_2 \rightarrow CaCO_3 + 2NaOH$

The reaction is exothermic and produces heat, sometimes up to 60 °C. One of the advantages of using low flow circle systems with soda lime is that the heat and water produced in the reaction help to warm and humidify the inspired gases. Soda lime is compatible with all the currently used volatile agents. Sevoflurane is degraded to Compound A in the presence of soda lime at elevated temperatures. While Compound A is nephrotoxic in rats there is no evidence of toxicity in humans. In the USA, however, sevoflurane is not licensed for use with soda lime at a fresh gas flow of less than 2 litres per minute. A danger recently highlighted by the Committee on Safety of Medicines (CSM) is the production of carbon monoxide when certain volatile agents react with dried out soda lime. This may then lead to carboxyhaemoglobinaemia in patients.

2.6 Sevoflurane **Answers: All false**

Sevoflurane is a fluorinated ether and is structurally related to enflurane and isoflurane, but is not an isomer of isoflurane. It is isoflurane and enflurane that are structural isomers of each other. Desflurane, another recently introduced volatile agent, requires a heated vaporiser, as its boiling point is 22.8 °C. While desflurane undergoes minimal metabolism (0.02%), sevoflurane undergoes about 5% metabolism. Sevoflurane is metabolised by the liver to produce inorganic fluoride ions. However, unlike enflurane, there is no evidence of renal toxicity from the fluoride ions produced by the metabolism of sevoflurane. Desflurane at > 1 MAC produces a degree of sympathetic stimulation with tachycardia and hypertension. Desflurane has a MAC of between 6 and 9%, while the MAC of sevoflurane is about 2%.

Ref: Anaesthetic Pharmacol. Rev. 1994: 2; 51–60.
Ref: BJA 1996: 76; 435–445.

2.7 Hypotension and elevated central venous pressure **Answers: A C D E**

In haemorrhage the central venous pressure (CVP) is low, as is the blood pressure, since there is a reduced intravascular volume. In all the other situations listed in the question there is either pump failure (myocardial infarction, congestive cardiac failure), or obstruction to the pulmonary circulation (pulmonary embolism, tension pneumothorax). In these instances therefore the damming back of blood in the venous circulation leads to an elevated CVP, while there is hypotension due to the pump failure or the obstruction to blood flow.

2.8 Adult VF arrest **Answers: B D**

The European Resuscitation Council issued guidelines for Advanced Life Support in 1992. They published algorithms for the management of VF/pulseless VT, EMD and asystole.

For adult VF arrest, the first shock should be 200 J. The next shock should also be 200 J and all subsequent shocks should be 360 J. The first drug to be given is adrenaline in a dose of 1 mg intravenously. Isoprenaline has no place in the management of VF arrest. It is used primarily in complete heart block while awaiting a tranvenous pacing wire. Intravenous bicarbonate is only considered after prolonged resuscitation, its use being guided by assessment of acid-base status. Bretylium tosylate, in a dose of 5–10 mg/kg may be considered where the VF has improved refractory to DC shocks.

2.9 Nimodipine **Answers: A C D**

Nimodipine is a calcium channel blocker (less correctly called a calcium antagonist). Like all calcium channel blockers, nimodipine causes vascular smooth muscle relaxation, and therefore can cause hypotension due to a reduction of systemic vascular resistance. Nimodipine, however, acts preferentially on cerebral arteries and its use is confined to prevention of vascular spasm following subarachnoid haemorrhage. It is not a cerebral protector per se, however.

2.10 Helium **Answers: A B**

Helium is stored as a gas at room temperature in brown cylinders at a pressure of 137 bar. It has a similar viscosity to oxygen, but is much less dense (density of oxygen is 1.3, helium 0.16). Its low density causes the voice changes seen when it is inhaled. Since density is an important determinant in turbulent flow, helium is useful in upper airway obstruction because of its low density, where flow is turbulent. It is, however, not of use in bronchospasm. Helium is non-flammable and does not support combustion.

2.11 Metabolic changes postoperatively **Answers: A B D E**

The metabolic and physiological changes that occur postoperatively are due in part to increased production of the stress hormones especially cortisol and the renin-angiotensin-aldosterone system. Cortisol antagonises the effects of insulin and causes hyperglycaemia. In addition it is catabolic and leads to protein breakdown and increased urinary nitrogen excretion. Both cortisol and aldosterone lead to retention of sodium coupled to increased urinary excretion of potassium. There is now much evidence to show that most patients experience quite profound sleep disturbances in the postoperative period.

2.12 Difficult intubation **Answers: A B C D**

There are many preoperative tests that are used to predict whether a patient is, or is not, likely to be difficult to intubate. Many of these tests yield a large number of false positives and, more worryingly, a significant number of false negatives too. Nevertheless a Mallampatti grade 3 does suggest a difficult intubation, as does a reduced thyromental distance. While obesity is associated with difficult intubation, there is no such association with Parkinson's disease. The Wilson score is made up of five variables: weight, head and neck movement, the presence or otherwise of buck teeth, a receding mandible, and mouth opening. Each variable is scored between 0–2 and a total score derived. A score of > 2 suggests a difficult intubation.

2.13 Massive blood transfusion **Answers: A B D**

There are several definitions of massive blood transfusion including the replacement of the patient's total blood volume by stored homologous bank blood in < 24 hours. One of the greatest problems is the inevitable developement of a coagulopathy, with thrombocytopenia and a prolonged international normalised ratio and activated partial thromboplastin time. This is readily corrected with FFP and platelets. Cryoprecipitate may be necessary if the fibrinogen level is very low. Disseminated intravascular coagulation (DIC) may occur in up to 30% of patients during a massive transfusion. Other problems with a massive transfusion include hypothermia, citrate toxicity, hypocalcaemia, hypokalaemia and a metabolic alkalosis. Pulmonary dysfunction may be caused by microaggregates in stored blood.

Ref: BJA 1992: 69; 621–630.

2.14 Acetylcholine **Answers: B D E**

Acetylcholine is the neurotransmitter at all autonomic ganglia, post-ganglionic parasympathetic nerve fibres and the neuromuscular junction. While noradrenaline is the neurotransmitter at most post-ganglionic sympathetic nerve fibres, the exception is the sweat glands. The adrenal medulla releases adrenaline and noradrenaline. The pre-ganglionic innervation of the adrenal medulla is cholinergic.

2.15 Constrictive pericarditis **Answers: A B E**

Constrictive pericarditis is characterised by a small heart on CXR, an elevated JVP, tachycardia, a low blood pressure and signs of right-sided heart failure. It may be due to tuberculosis, carcinoma, radiotherapy, rheumatoid arthritis or trauma. Usually there is an elevated JVP and ascites but no pulmonary oedema. There is pulsus paradoxus (an exaggerated fall in blood pressure on inspiration). The elevated JVP rises further on inspiration (Kussmaul's sign) and exhibits a rapid descent.

2.16 Aortic regurgitation **Answers: A B C D E**

The causes of aortic regurgitation are rheumatic fever, rheumatoid arthritis, bacterial endocarditis, hypertension, dissecting aortic aneurysm, syphilis, Marfan's syndrome, and the seronegative arthropathies including ankylosing spondylitis, Reiter's syndrome, psoriatic arthropathy and relapsing polychondritis.

2.17 Acute spinal cord injury **Answers: B D**

In acute spinal cord injury, suxamethonium is safe if given within 72 hours of the injury. Steroids may be of some benefit in acute cord injury. There is usually hypotension and bradycardia due to loss of the sympathetic innervation. Hypotension is undesirable as it reduces blood supply to an already compromised spinal cord.

2.18 Autonomic neuropathy **Answers: A C**

Autonomic neuropathy is most commonly seen in diabetes mellitus, but can occur in AIDS, the Shy Drager syndrome (a variant of Parkinson's disease), and with bronchial carcinoma. The Valsalva manoeuvre is a standard test of the integrity of the autonomic nervous system (ANS). In ANS dysfunction there is no variation in heart rate during the test. Normally there is a variation in heart rate with respiration; this is absent in ANS dysfunction. This can be demonstrated either on the ECG or by simple palpation of the peripheral pulse. Postural hypotension occurs in ANS dysfunction.

2.19 Deep vein thrombosis **Answers: A B C D E**

DVT occurs commonly in the postoperative period. Pulmonary embolism, which may follow on from DVT remains a common cause of post operative death. The likelihood of developing a DVT is increased by the oral contraceptive pill. Pregnancy also increases the likelihood. Despite its name, the lupus anticoagulant is associated with an increased chance of developing a DVT. HbSC disease is particularly associated with DVT, especially during pregnancy. Polycythaemia and the other myeloproliferative disorders predispose to DVT.

2.20 Myxoedema coma **Answers: A C D E**

Myxoedema coma is a medical emergency; mortality is about 50%. A patient with myxoedema coma looks hypothyriod, is hypothermic, hyporeflexic, bradycardic and comatose. Treatment should be in an intensive care unit and includes intravenous thyroxine (T4) or triiodothyronine (T3) as a bolus and then regularly for 2–3 days. If pituitary hypothyroidism is suspected then intravenous hydrocortiosone is given to replace ACTH deficiency. Hypothermia is very common and requires active rewarming. Hypothermia can lead to pancreatitis, hypoglycaemia and ventricular fibrillation. Thyroxine (T4) is given orally once the patient is stabilised. Either normal saline or dextrose can be given; the latter is used if there is hypoglycaemia.

2.21 Acromegaly **Answers: A B D E**

Acromegaly is due to hypersecretion of growth hormone from a pituitary tumour. Patients have coarse oily skin, prognathism, and a large tongue. Arthralgia, glucose intolerance, hypertension and a thyroid goitre may occur. Hyperprolactinaemia may occur, leading to impotence, galacto-rrhoea, gynaecomastia and amenorrhoea in females. There may be hypercalcaemia and hyperphosphataemia with a tendency to form renal calculi. Progresive heart failure may be seen.

2.22 Diabetic autonomic neuropathy **Answers: A B C D E**

Diabetic patients are at increased risk of preoperative complications, mainly from autonomic nervous system (ANS) dysfunction. ANS dys-function is asociated with increased cardiovascular instability during anaesthesia. These patients generally fail to exhibit the usual pressor response to tracheal intubation and have a prolonged QT interval. Profound hypotension, bradycardia and even asystole may occur during anaesthesia. Impotence, diarrhoea, incomplete bladder emptying and loss of sweat in the limbs are other manifestations of ANS dysfunction that may occur.

Ref: Curr Opinion Anaesthesiol 1996: 9; 247–253.

2.23 Bleeding time **Answers: B C E**

The bleeding time is essentially a test of platelet and vascular function. Vitamin K is required by the liver for the synthesis of clotting factors 2, 7, 9 and 10. A deficiency of this vitamin leads to a prolongation of both PT and APTT, but has no effect on the bleeding time. Scurvy, due to deficiency of vitamin C, however, does prolong the bleeding time. This is because vitamin C is required for collagen synthesis. The defective collagen in the blood vessels in scurvy leads to a prolonged bleeding time. Haemophilia A and von Willebrand's disease are both inherited disorders affecting clotting factor 8. Factor 8 consists of several subunits. In haemophilia A, factor 8c is deficient, leading to a prolongation of the APTT. In von Willebrand's disease, factor 8VWF is abnormal. Since this part of the factor 8 molecule is needed for platelet adhesion the bleeding time is also prolonged in addition to the APTT. In DIC there is consumption of clotting factors and platelets, leading to prolongation of PT, APTT and bleeding time.

2.24 Antibiotic cover for patients with prosthetic heart valve **Answers: B C**

The British National Formulary (BNF) contains guidelines for prophylaxis against endocarditis in patients with prosthetic heart valves. A patient with a prosthetic heart valve having dental work is considered high risk and must receive antibiotic cover. The BNF recommends IM/IV amoxycillin 1 g and IM/IV gentamicin 120 mg at induction; then oral amoxycillin 500 mg 6 hours later. Patients who are penicillin allergic may have either vancomycin and gentamicin or teicoplanin and gentamicin or clindamycin alone.

2.25 Teratogens **Answers: A B E**

A teratogen is an agent that causes structural or functional abnormalities in the fetus, or in the child after birth. The most commonly recognised teratogens include thalidomide, the androgens, cytotoxics, lithium, retinoids and warfarin. Lithium can cause a hypotonic baby and in addition is associated with atrialisation of the tricuspid valve (Ebstein's anomaly). Warfarin should be avoided in the first trimester, when heparin should be used instead. Warfarin can be re-instituted from week 12. Warfarin can cause fetal asplenia, rendering the neonate susceptible to infection with *Pneumococcus* and other organisms. It can also cause chondrodysplasia punctata. Carbamazepine may be associated with neural tube defects. None of the inhalational anaesthetic agents are teratogens. Although the tetracyclines can cause staining of the teeth in the developing fetus, they are not teratogens.

2.26 TUR syndrome **Answers: A B E**

The TUR syndrome may occur as a result of absorption of the irrigating fluid used. The volume absorbed is reduced if the height of the irrigating fluid is < 60 cm, duration of surgery < 60 min. About 20 ml/hr is normally absorbed. The fluid used is iso-osmotic 1.5% glycine solution. As it is iso-osmotic its absorption does not cause haemolysis. Glycine is used as it has good optical properties without conducting electricity, thereby reducing the risk of burns. Glycine is an inhibitory neurotransmitter and thus its absorption causes CNS effects such as confusion, seizures, cerebral oedema and irritability. Absorption of large volumes of irrigating fluid into the vascular space leads to signs of pulmonary oedema and heart failure, often with hypotension and, paradoxically, bradycardia. Classically there is hyponatraemia due to dilution. The management involves giving oxygen, fluid restriction and possibly a diuretic. The serum sodium must be corrected slowly as too rapid correction may lead to central pontine myelinolysis, which has a very high mortality. Disseminated intravascular coagulation can occur as part of the TUR syndrome.

2.27 Ropivacaine **Answers: A B E**

Ropivacaine is a new amide local anaesthetic agent. It is slightly less potent than bupivacaine, but has a similar duration of action. Its main advantages are that it has less central nervous and cardiovascular toxicity than bupivacaine and is more selective for sensory nerve fibres. Unlike bupivacaine, which is a racemic mixture, ropivacaine is a single enantiomer. Plasma protein binding of ropivacaine is slightly less than that of bupivacaine but the pKa is identical.

Ref: BJA 1996: 76; 300–307.

2.28 Fat embolism **Answers: A B C D E**

Fat embolism occurs with fracture or operation on a long bone. A triad of respiratory compromise, cerebral dysfunction and petechial haemorrhages may be seen. There may be a pyrexia and ARDS or DIC can supervene in severe cases. It is associated with a mortality of 10–20%.

2.29 Recurrent laryngeal nerve **Answers: A B C**

The innervation of the larynx is derived from the superior and recurrent laryngeal branches of the vagus nerve.

The recurrent laryngeal nerve supplies:

1. Sensory fibres to the larynx below the vocal cords.
2. Motor fibres to all the intrinsic muscles of the larynx, except cricothyroid.

The superior laryngeal nerve supplies:

1. Sensory fibres to the larynx above the vocal cords.
2. Motor fibres to cricothyroid.

The recurrent laryngeal nerves are intimately related to the inferior thyroid arteries.

2.30 Convulsions **Answers: A C D**

There are many causes of convulsions that may affect the anaesthetist. Among these are the metabolic causes such as hypoglycaemia, hypocalcaemia, hypomagnesaemia and hyponatraemia. Alcohol withdrawl, renal or hepatic disease and drug poisoning are all potential causes. Head injuries or intracranial pathology may be implicated. Anaesthetic drugs including enflurane may be the aetiology. Hypoxia is a potent trigger for convulsions.

2.31 Primary hyperparathyroidism **Answers: A B C E**

Primary hyperparathyroidism is most commonly caused by an adenoma of the parathyroid glands. It leads to demineralisation of bones with extraosseous calcification, increased plasma and urinary calcium and renal calculi.

2.32 Lower oesophageal tone **Answers: A C**

Metaclopramide and cisapride are pro-kinetic drugs and promote gastric emptying. However metaclopramide is, in addition, an anti-emetic and increases lower oesophageal sphincter (LOS) tone. Atropine and morphine both reduce LOS tone. Domperidone is, like metaclopramide an antagonist at dopaminergic receptors. It also increases LOS tone.

2.33 Magnesium **Answers: A B C D E**

Magnesium has a number of properties that are relevant to anaesthesia. It has effects at the neuromuscular junction, the CNS, the myocardium and peripheral vascular tree. It sits in the central core of the NMDA receptor. It is used as an anticonvulsant in eclampsia, as an antiarrythmic and in the treatment of phaeochromocytoma. Hypomagnesaemia is seen in alcoholics, diabetic ketoacidosis and in patients taking digoxin or diuretics. It can cause tetany, seizures and prolongation of the QT interval leading to VT or torsades de pointes. Hypermagnesaemia is seen in Addison's disease, chronic renal failure and in patients on lithium therapy. Magnesium readily crosses the placenta and may lead to fetal hypotonia and respiratory depression. Magnesium inhibits acetylcholine release from the neuromuscular junction and so potentiates the actions of the non-depolarising muscle relaxants.

Ref: International Journal of Obstetric Anaesthesia 1998: 7; 115–123.

2.34 Alfentanil **Answer: D**

Compared with fentanyl, alfentanil has a greater pKa. Alfentanil is more lipid-soluble and faster acting, but less potent. Alfentanil has a smaller volume of distribution and a more rapid elimination. It has no active metabolites.

2.35 Radial nerve palsy **Answers: A B D**

The radial nerve supplies triceps, brachioradialis and extensor carpi radialis longus. Hence damage to the nerve leads to paralysis of the extensor muscles of the forearm and hand, causing wrist drop. Pronation is a function of pronater teres, innervated by the median nerve. It is supination which is affected by radial nerve palsy. Because of nerve overlap there is usually only a small area of anaesthesia in a radial nerve palsy, confined to the base of the thumb. The thenar eminence is innervated by the median nerve.

2.36 Papilloedema **Answers: A B C D**

Papilloedema is due to raised intracranial pressure. It is usually due to a space occupying lesion such as a cerebral tumour or abscess. It can rarely be seen in cavernous sinus thrombosis, and with both occlusion of the central retinal artery and vein. It can be unilateral, as in the Foster Kennedy syndrome.There is optic atrophy in one eye, papilloedema in the other. It is caused by a tumour on the inferior surface of the contralateral frontal lobe. It can be seen with the hypercapnia of respiratory failure. However, in respiratory failure due to pulmonary oedema the $PaCO_2$ is not usually elevated.

2.37 Non-steroidal anti-inflammatory drugs (NSAIDs) **Answers: A B D E**

The NSAIDs act by inhibiting the enzyme cyclo-oxygenase which is involved in prostaglandin synthesis. Prostaglandins sensitise peripheral nociceptors to the effects of substance P, histamine and serotonin. By blocking prostaglandin synthesis, the NSAIDs are analgesic. Prostaglandins are a group of compounds derived from arachidonic acid. Arachidonic acid may be converted by the enzyme lipo-oxygenase to leukotrienes most of which are bronchoconstrictors. Alternatively arachidonic acid may be converted by cyclo-oxygenase to cyclic endoperoxides and thence to either thromboxane (TXA2) or prostacyclin (PGI2). TXA2 is produced by platelet cyclo-oxygenase and is a potent vasoconstrictor and platelet agggregator. PGI2 is produced by vascular endothelium and is a vasodilator. In about 10% of asthmatics, especially those with atopic asthma, allergic rhinitis and nasal polyps, NSAIDs may precipitate bronchospasm. This may be due to the unopposed bronchoconstrictor action of the leukotrienes. NSAIDs may precipitate acute renal failure especially in elderly, dehydrated patients.

Prostaglandins are vasodilators at the renal afferent arteriole and thus NSAIDs may cause vasoconstriction, ischaemia and acute tubular necrosis. By blockade of TXA2, NSAIDS inhibit platelet aggregation and may exacerbate surgical blood loss. In the gastric mucosa, prostaglandins have a cytoprotective effect and NSAIDs may cause gastric inhibition, peptic ulceration and even gastrointestinal haemorrhage or perforation. NSAIDs may be given with misoprostol, a synthetic prostaglandin to prevent this side-effect.
There are in fact two types of cyclo-oxygenase; COX-1 and COX-2. The COX-1 enzyme is protective and it is blockage of this that produces renal failure, platelet dysfunction and gastrointestinal bleeding. By selectively blocking COX-2 these side-effects are, in theory at least, avoided. Although meloxicam is the only COX-2 selective NSAID on the market, diclofenac is relatively COX-2 selective.

Ref: Royal College of Anaesthetists, Jan 1998. Guidelines for the use of non-steroidal anti-inflammatory drugs in the peri-operative period.

2.38 Respiratory support **Answers: A B C D E**

A patient who is tired and sweating, with bounding peripheral pulses may well be in hypercarbic respiratory failure and require respiratory support. Use of the accessory muscles of respiration and a tracheal tug also suggest the patient is becoming exhausted and will require respiratory support.

2.39 Brain stem death **Answers: D E**

Before performing tests of brain stem function, two preconditions must be met:

1. The presence of apnoeic coma.
2. Irreversible brain damage of known aetiology.

Potentially reversible conditions that may mimic brain stem death (BSD) must be excluded, such as:

1. Alcohol, sedatives, muscle relaxants, poisons.
2. Hypothermia; the temperature must be > 35 °C.
3. Acid-base disturbance.
4. Endocrine or metabolic disturbance; hypothyroidism or thyrotoxicosis, diabetic coma (either hypo- or hyper-glycaemia), hyponatraemia.

BSD is confirmed by the demonstration of the absence of brain stem reflexes. This must be performed by two doctors: one should be the patient's consultant. Both must be medically registered for > 5 years; neither should be a member of the transplant team.

The tests are:
1. Fixed unresponsive pupils (pupil size is irrelevant).
2. Absent corneal reflexes.
3. Absent doll's eye movements, (i.e. the eyes do not move relative to the orbit when the head is rotated side to side).
4. Absence of gag reflex.
5. Absence of vestibulo-ocular reflexes.
6. Absence of motor activity within the cranial nerve territory after painful stimuli to the head and peripherally. Limb movement may occur but is due to spinal reflexes and does not exclude the diagnosis of BSD.
7. Absence of spontaneous respiratory effort. During this test the $PaCO_2$ must be > 6.7 kPa (i.e. sufficient to stimulate breathing). Patients with chronic lung disease who rely on hypoxic drive should have a PaO_2 of < 6.7 kPa.

2.40 Pulse oximeter **Answers: A B E**

The pulse oximeter is used to measure the saturation of haemoglobin with oxygen. It is not a good monitor of ventilatory adequacy, especially in the context of a patient breathing at high inspired oxygen tension. The other limitations to its use include the fact that both motion and ambient light may cause erroneous readings. Both methaemoglobin and carboxyhaemoglobin produce false readings, but the pulse oximeter is perfectly accurate in the presence of HbF, as in the neonate. The pulse oximeter is accurate in dark-skinned patients, but may be inaccurate in the presence of intense vasoconstriction.

Ref: BMJ 1993: 307; 457–458.
Ref: BMJ 1995: 311; 367–370.

2.41 Cushing's syndrome **Answers: A B D E**

Cushing's syndrome leads to hypokalaemia and a metabolic alkalosis. A gastrocolic fistula leads to loss of gastric acid, as does pyloric stenosis. Acetazolamide is a carbonic anhydrase inhibitor which may be used to treat metabolic alkalosis.

2.42 Trigeminal neuralgia **Answers: B C D E**

Trigeminal neuralgia affects the 5th cranial nerve. It may be treated with carbamazepine, but may be intractable. It may, rarely, be a presenting feature in multiple sclerosis.

2.43 Arterial line in the radial artery **Answers: A B C D E**

All of the options are potential complications of the siting of an arterial line.

2.44 Exponential process **Answers: B C E**

The half-life is the time taken for the quantity of whatever is being measured to fall to half of its original value. The time constant is the time at which the process would have been complete had the initial rate of change been maintained. The time constant is longer than the half-life. After one time constant the original quantity has fallen to 37% of its original value and after three time constants 95% of the process is completed.

2.45 Cervical cord injury **Answers: A B C D**

The combination of hypotension and bradycardia suggests neurogenic shock and is due to loss of sympathetic vasomotor tone and the cardioaccelerator fibres. Although ultimately there will be signs of spasticity, due to upper motor neurone damage, initially there is spinal shock. Spinal shock is manifest as are flexic flaccidity of the limbs. Damage to the phrenic nerve (C3, 4, 5) occurs with high cervical cord injuries and leads to paralysis of the diaphragm. Lower lesions may only affect the intercostal muscles with less respiratory impairment.

2.46 Etomidate **Answers: A B C D E**

Etomidate is a carboxylated imidazole. It is soluble, but stable, in water and therefore presented in 35% propylene glycol. It is eliminated by esterase hydrolysis in the liver and plasma. Etomidate depresses the synthesis of both cortisol and aldosterone by inhibition of the adrenal enzyme, 11 beta hydroxylase. It has a low incidence of allergy and does not cause histamine release. It causes pain on injection, involuntary movements and there is a high incidence of post-operative nausea and vomiting. It is porphyrinogenic in animal models and is therefore probably best avoided in known porphyric patients.

2.47 Malignant hyperpyrexia **Answers: A B C E**

Malignant hyperpyrexia is inherited as an autosomal dominant gene.The disease affects skeletal muscle and is characterised by episodes of muscle hypermetabolism. It may be precipitated by a number of anaesthetic drugs including, classically, halothane and suxamethonium. The local anaesthetic agents are all safe. Although previously thought to be associated with other muscle disorders such as Duchenne muscular dystrophy the only definite association is with central core disease. The disease is thought to be due to an abnormality of the ryanodine receptor which is the calcium channel in the sarcoplasmic reticulum of the muscle. Uncontrolled entry of calcium into the muscle leads to hyperpyrexia and muscle rigidity. The muscle damage that ensues leads to rhabdomyolysis, hyperkalaemia and acidosis. The only specific treatment is dantrolene. Diagnosis is by in vitro contracture tests on muscle using halothane and caffeine.

Ref: Current Anaesthesia & Critical Care 1996: 6; 87–94.
Ref: Anaesthesiology 1996: 84; 1275–1279.

2.48 Air embolism **Answers: A B**

Air embolism may occur during posterior fossa surgery. It is detected by a sudden fall in end-tidal carbon dioxide on capnography. The treatment includes turning off the nitrous oxide and giving 100% oxygen. Nitrous oxide is much less soluble than nitrogen and will increase the size of an air embolism. Mannitol will help reduce cerebral oedema but is of no value in air embolism. Compression of the neck veins elevates the venous pressure and together with flooding of the surgical site with saline, prevents further air entering the circulation. Lying the patient head down in the left lateral position keeps the air embolism away from the pulmonary artery and coronary ostium, by trapping it in the right ventricle.

2.49 Amniotic fluid embolism **Answers: A B C D E**

If amniotic fluid enters the circulation it produces sudden severe shock with respiratory distress and cyanosis. There is usually a raised CVP and widespread opacification of the lung fields. ARDS may develop. There is often a coagulopathy, usually DIC. The mortality rate is very high. Treatment is supportive. A definitive diagnosis is usually made at post mortem, although fetal squames may be found in pulmonary artery blood if a pulmonary artery catheter is in place. There is some evidence that the more forceful uterine contractions are, as occurs with syntocinon infusion, the more likely amniotic fluid embolism is.

2.50 Cardioplegia **Answers: B C D E**

Cardioplegia is used for myocardial preservation while the aorta is cross clamped during cardiac surgery. Potassium is present in a concentration of 10–20 mmol/l. It causes depolarisation of the myocardial cells and arrest in diastole. Procaine is present as a membrane stabiliser, while magnesium reduces automatic rhythmogenicity.

2.51 Ankle block **Answers: B D E**

There are five nerves to be blocked in an ankle block; tibial, sural, saphenous, deep and superficial peroneal nerves. Apart from the saphenous nerve, which is a branch of the femoral, all the other nerves are derived from the sciatic. The tibial nerve lies behind the medial malleolus and deep to the posterior tibial artery. The sural nerve lies between the Achilles tendon and lateral malleolus. The saphenous nerve lies anterior to the medial malleolus. The superficial peroneal nerve lies above and medial to the lateral malleolus. The deep peroneal nerve lies between extensor hallucis longus and tibialis anterior and is lateral to the anterior tibial artery.

2.52 Disseminated intravascular coagulation (DIC) **Answers: A B C D**

DIC is a consumptive coagulopathy that may be triggered by many disorders. The result is consumption of platelets, fibrinogen and clotting factors with, paradoxically, widespread deposition of thrombus in the microvasculature of vital organs such as the kidney and brain. This thrombus activates thrombolysis and perpetuates the coagulopathy. The management, in essence, entails replacing what is missing i.e. platelets, fibrinogen (cryoprecipitate) and clotting factors (FFP). Of relevance to the anaesthetist is the fact that it may occur in several obstetric situations including severe pre eclampsia or eclampsia, amniotic fluid embolus and placental abruption. It may occur with haemolytic transfusion reactions, following prostatectomy and in any septic patient.

Ref: BMJ 1996: 312; 683–687.

2.53 Acute liver failure **Answers: B C D E**

Acute liver failure may be due to viral hepatitis (hepatitis A, B, C, CMV or EBV), alcohol, paracetamol or other toxins and, rarely, halothane. The commonest cause in the UK is paracetamol overdose. Indicators of a poor prognosis include a prothrombin time > 3x control, bilirubin > 300 micromol/l and a pH < 7.3. The liver enzymes alanine and aspartate aminotransferase (ALT, AST) are characteristically elevated and are sensitive markers of hepatocellular damage.

2.54 Complications of tracheostomy **Answers: A B C D E**

The complications of tracheostomy may be early or late.

Early:

1. Bleeding
2. Pneumothorax
3. Cardiovascular collapse if hypoxia or respiratory acidosis is rapidly corrected.

Late:
1. Infection
2. Tracheal stenosis
3. Erosion into cartilage, major vessel or oesophagus
4. Obstruction of tracheostomy tube.

2.55 Blood cell antigen A **Answers: A C E**

The ABO blood groups are inherited in Mendelian fashion.

The ABO blood group system

Phenotype	Genotype	Antigens	Naturally occurring antibodies	Frequency (%)
O	OO	O	Anti-A, B	46
A	AA or AO	A	Anti-B	42
B	BB or BO	B	Anti-A	9
AB	AB	AB	None	3

O is universal donor
AB is universal recipient

The table shows the frequency of each blood type. The ABO blood group antigens are found on red cells, white cells and platelets and in the 80% of the population who possess secretor genes, they are also found in saliva, plasma, semen and sweat. Haemolytic disease of the newborn (HDN) is the result of damage to fetal cells by maternal IgG antibodies directed against fetal red cell antigens. Until recently HDN was almost always due to anti-D antibodies produced by a rhesus-negative mother who was carrying a fetus with rhesus-positive red cells. Since the introduction of prophylactic anti-D for rhesus-negative mothers the incidence of HDN has fallen dramatically and of the few cases that do occur most commonly it is due to anti-A produced by a mother of group O against the red cells of a group A fetus.

2.56 Left ventricular failure (LVF) **Answer: B D E**

The pulmonary oedema of left ventricular failure (LVF) can often clinically resemble asthma. Both produce dyspnoea and wheeziness. LVF is more likely to cause a elevated jugular venous pressure (JVP). LVF is associated with pulsus alternans while asthma causes pulsus paradoxus. Both will cause hypoxia and resulting cyanosis. Both can cause wheeze on auscultation of the lung fields, but the wheeze is expiratory in asthma while there are classically fine, basal, inspiratory crepitations in LVF. While pulmonary oedema of LVF produces bilateral fluffy infiltration on the chest X-ray there are usually clear lung fields in the asthmatic's CXR.

2.57 Obstructive lung disease **Answers: B C**

Obstructive lung disease (e.g. asthma) is characterised by a reduced FEV1/FVC ratio and a reduced PEFR. Restrictive lung disease is characterised by a reduction in both FEV1 and FRC resulting in a normal ratio.The TLCO is reduced.

2.58 Erythropoietin **Answers: A C**

Erythropoietin is made in the kidneys (85%) and the liver (15%). It promotes red cell production by the bone marrow. Production is stimulated by hypoxia or haemorrhage. Production is reduced in renal disease and accounts, in part, for the anaemia of chronic renal failure.

2.59 Oxyhaemoglobin dissociation curve **Answers: A B**

The oxyhaemoglobin dissociation curve position depends critically on the plasma concentration of 2,3 DPG. The P75 represents the oxygen partial pressure at which haemoglobin is 75% saturated with oxygen, i.e. venous blood. This is normally about 5.3 kPa (40 mmHg). The curve is shifted to the right (the Bohr effect) by decreased pH, raised temperature, raised levels of 2,3 DPG (as in chronic anaemia), altitude and hypoxia. The curve shifts to the left in carbon monoxide poisoning, in the presence of HbF or other high affinity haemoglobins. A rightward shift of the curve enables the tissues to extract oxygen from haemoglobin more easily.

2.60 Rheumatoid arthritis **Answers: A C D E**

Rheumatoid arthritis is a systemic chronic inflammatory disease affecting up to 3% of women and 1% of men in the United Kingdom. Although the brunt of the disease is borne by the joints, most of the organs are affected. In the cardiovascular system the pericardium, myocardium and endocardium may all be affected. There is often a normochromic normocytic anaemia. Renal failure may be due to analgesic nephropathy, amyloidosis or an autoimmune glomerulonephritis.

Ref: Anaesthesia 1993: 48; 989–997.

2.61 Neonatal airway **Answers: A C D E**

The trachea is 4 cm long in the neonate; the narrowest part is the cricoid cartilage. The larynx is at C4 and reaches the adult position (opposite C5/6) at 4 years old. The epiglottis is U-shaped and the tracheal rings are not fully formed. The carina is at T2 (T4 in the adult).

2.62 Fallot's tetralogy **Answers: A B**

Fallot's tetralogy accounts for 10% of all congenital heart disease and 50% of cyanotic congenital heart disease. It consists of a VSD, pulmonary stenosis, right ventricular hypertrophy and an overriding aorta. Clinical signs include clubbing and cyanosis and a murmur due to flow across the stenosed pulmonary valve. Syncope and squatting are often seen.

2.63 Hypofibrinogenaemia **Answers: A C D E**

In massive transfusion the level of platelets and clotting factors is reduced as stored blood contains no effective platelets and is deficient in clotting factors, including fibrinogen. A similar situation exists in disseminated intravascular coagulation (DIC) although the aetiology is entirely different. The oral contraceptive pill leads to an increase in fibrinogen, a hypercoagulable state and an increased incidence of venous thromboembolism. Asparaginase, used in the treatment of childhood acute lymphoblastic leukaemia causes hypofibrinogenaemia. Prostate resection may lead to the release of procoagulant material into the circulation and a resulting consumptive coagulopathy.

2.64 Morphine **Answers: A B D E**

Morphine is an agonist at mu and kappa opioid receptors. The mu receptors are further subdivided into mu1 and mu2. Stimulation of mu1 receptors leads to analgesia. Stimulation of mu2 receptors leads to euphoria, ventilatory depression and miosis (by stimulation of the Edinger-Westphal nucleus of the 3rd cranial nerve), bradycardia, inappropriate ADH release and reduced gastrointestinal motility. Morphine can cause histamine release and nausea and vomiting (by stimulation of the chemoreceptor trigger zone). Morphine is metabolised in the liver to morphine-6-glucuronide; itself a potent analgesic, devoid of some of the unwanted side-effects of morphine.

2.65 Retrobulbar block **Answers: All false**

In a retrobulbar block, local anaesthetic is injected into the muscle cone thereby anaesthetising the ciliary nerves, ciliary ganglion, 3rd and 6th cranial nerves. A separate facial nerve block is required to paralyse the obicularis oculi muscle. The lacrimal nerve, which controls lacrimation, sits outside the muscle cone and is not affected by a retrobulbar block. Enophthalmos and miosis are part of Horner's syndrome, due to loss of the cervical sympathetic supply to the eye.This is seen in a stellate ganglion block, not in retrobulbar anaesthesia. Although the intraocular pressure usually increases with a retrobulbar block, there is no rise in intracranial pressure and thus no papilloedema.

Ref: Br J Hosp Med 1993: 49; 689–701.
Ref: BJA 1995: 75; 80–95.

2.66 Phaeochromocytomata **Answers: A B C D**

Phaeochromocytomata are the tumour of 10s:10% are bilateral, 10% are familial, 10% are malignant. The familial tumours may be associated with hyperparathyroidism, medullary thyroid cancer and pancreatic or pituitary tumours. They may secrete adrenaline, noradrenaline, dopamine, somatostatin and other neuropeptides. They may cause continuous or episodic hypertension, or hypotension. The adrenaline secretion causes hyperglycaemia.

2.67 Myaesthenia gravis **Answers: B D**

Myaesthenia is an autoimmune disease characterised by a high titre of antibodies directed against the post-synaptic acetylcholine receptor of the neuromuscular junction. It is often associated with a thymoma. Oat cell tumours are associated with the Eaton-Lambert syndrome. Myaesthenia may be treated by thymectomy, immunosuppression, plasmaphaeresis and anticholinesterases. There is increased sensitivity to non-depolarising muscle relaxants.

2.68 Mitral stenosis **Answers: A B D E**

Mitral stenosis is associated with a loud first heart sound, an opening snap and a low pitched rumbling mid-diastolic murmur heard best at the apex with the patient lying in the left lateral postion. Atrial fibrillation is common in mitral valve disease.The patient often has a malar flush. The apex beat is tapping in quality, but is not displaced.

2.69 Post abdominal surgery – complications **Answers: B D**

The patient is febrile, shocked (low BP and tachycardia) and has a low CVP. The likeliest explanation is that the patient is septic, which may be due to anastomotic breakdown. Although tachycardia and hypotension are seen in myocardial infarction and cardiac tamponade there is no pyrexia and the CVP is usually elevated.

2.70 Coronary artery blood flow **Answers: A B C D**

Coronary artery blood flow occurs mainly in diastole. As heart rate increases the length of diastole decreases and thus tachycardia reduces coronary blood flow. If venous pressure rises the left ventricular end diastolic pressure rises and myocardial wall tension increases leading to reduced coronary blood flow. Coronary artery blood flow is autoregulated and controlled by local mediators such as hydrogen ions, potassium ions and nitric oxide. Blood flow is increased by hypoxia.

2.71 Tidal volume increase **Answers: B E**

An increase in tidal volume is seen in renal failure and diabetic ketoacidosis. It is a physiological response to acidosis and is mediated by the peripheral chemoreceptors, located in the aortic and carotid bodies. Ankylosing spondylitis is associated with a reduced tidal volume and a restrictive lung defect. Cerebral haemorrhage usually causes respiratory depression.

2.72 Specific gravity of urine **Answers: A B D**

Diabetes insipidus (which may occur with lithium toxicity) leads to the production of large amounts of dilute urine, as the renal tubules either fail to respond to ADH or the posterior pituitary fails to produce ADH. In diabetes mellitus the glucose in the urine raises its specific gravity. In intestinal obstruction the resulting dehydration causes oliguria and the production of small amounts of concentrated urine, while in acute tubular necrosis small amounts of poor quality urine are produced.

2.73 Microshock **Answers: A C**

Microshock is the term used to describe the delivery of very small currents (100–150 microamps) directly to the myocardium, where they may cause ventricular fibrillation. (VF) Microshock requires the presence of a faulty intracardiac catheter (e.g. CVP line) or pacemaker electrode touching the wall of the heart along which current can pass.

Saline-filled intracardiac catheters will conduct current, while 5% dextrose will reduce the hazard of microshock.

The severity of microshock is inversely related to current frequency so risk is greatest at low frequencies such as mains frequency and with direct current. Connecting intracardiac catheters to isolated (floating, non-earthed) power supplies reduces the risk of microshock.

Ref: Basic Physics and Measurement in Anaesthetics by Parbrook and Parbrook 3rd edition, Butterworth Heinemann; 213-215.

2.74 The blood-brain barrier (BBB) **Answers: A B E**

The blood-brain barrier (BBB) forms a barrier between the cerebral circulation and the brain tissue. Lipid-soluble drugs such as fentanyl rapidly cross the BBB. Highly ionised drugs such as the quaternary amine neostigmine cannot cross. Tertiary amines, however, such as atropine and hyoscine, do cross the BBB. L-Dopa crosses the BBB where it is converted to dopamine which does not cross. Mannitol is given to treat cerebral oedema. As it does not normally cross the BBB it acts as an osmotic diuretic and draws water across the BBB and into the vascular space by osmosis.

2.75 Speed of uptake of an anaesthetic agent **Answer: B**

The speed of uptake of an anaesthetic agent is proportional to the minute ventilation and inversely proportional to the cardiac output and the blood gas solubility coefficient. It is unrelated to the MAC and is not temperature dependent.

2.76 Diabetic amyotrophy **Answers: B C**

Diabetic amyotrophy is a form of somatic neuropathy which causes wasting (usually of the quadriceps) and pain in the affected muscles. It is associated with an elevated CSF protein and responds to improved blood sugar control. Impotence and urinary retention in the diabetic may signify autonomic neuropathy.

2.77 Ruptured oesophagus **Answer: D**

The most likely diagnosis here is a ruptured oesophagus (Boerhaave's syndrome). This is usually caused by excessive vomiting. The patient complains of epigastric pain and there is surgical emphysema in the neck. Pulmonary infarction would produce chest pains and laboured breathing but no subcutaneous emphysema or epigastric guarding. Similarly pneumothorax and ruptured trachea do not produce epigastric guarding. A ruptured diaphragm tends to produce shoulder tip pain as its innervation is from C3–C5.

2.78 Dystrophia myotonica **Answers: A C D E**

Inherited as an autosomal dominant gene, this condition, though rare, has implications for anaesthesia. The myotonia (delayed muscle relaxation following contraction) affects skeletal and smooth muscle. It may be precipitated by cold, shivering and suxamethonium and neostigmine. Patients may have frontal balding with wasting of the sternocleidomastoid and temporalis. The disease is associated with low IQ, diabetes mellitus, gonadal atrophy, dysphagia, respiratory muscle failure and a cardiomypathy. There is increased sensitivity to non-depolarising muscle relaxants and extreme sensitivity to opioids, barbiturates and volatile agents.

Ref: BJA 1994: 72; 210–216.

2.79 Brown-Sequard syndrome **Answers: B C D E**

The Brown-Sequard syndrome is due to hemisection of the spinal cord. There is ipsilateral spastic paralysis (upper motor neurone lesion) with contralateral analgesia and thermoanaesthesia due to destruction of the spinothalamic tract. Damage to the dorsal columns produces ipsilateral loss of vibration and joint position awareness and Rombergism.

2.80 Vomiting **Answers: A B E**

Vomiting leads to loss of HCl from the stomach, leading to a metabolic alkalosis. The resulting dehydration causes a raised blood urea. The kidney attempts to compensate by conserving hydrogen ions in exchange for potassium, hence the alkaline urine and low plasma potassium.

2.81 Crohn's disease **Answers: A B C E**

Crohn's is a granulomatous condition affecting the bowel. It is associated with fistulae and perianal sepsis. Arthritis, uveitis and skin rashes may occur. Lymphoma is associated with coeliac disease.

2.82 Glycosuria **Answers: A B E**

Glycosuria occurs commonly in pregnancy. It is found in subarachnoid haemorrhage and phaeochromocytoma due to the high levels of circulating catecholamines. Hypopituitarism and partial gastrectomy are causes of hypoglycaemia.

2.83 Cardiac tamponade **Answers: A B C**

Cardiac tamponade is associated with an elevated JVP and a reduced cardiac output. The radial pulse is weak and becomes even weaker on inspiration, so called pulsus paradoxus. It may be differentiated from CCF as it is associated with a small heart on CXR, little or no pulmonary oedema, and hepatomegaly and ascites. It requires pericardiocentesis or surgery.

2.84 Electrocardiography **Answers: A E**

At rest the interior of the cell is negatively charged with respect to the exterior. This is due to an unequal ion distribution across the cell membrane, with potassium being mainly an intracellular ion and sodium being predominantly extracellular. The PR interval is prolonged in first degree heart block and the QT interval is prolonged in hypocalcaemia.

2.85 Ketamine **Answers: C D E**

Ketamine is a phencyclidine derivative, presented as a racemic mixture. It produces a unique state of dissociative anaesthesia. It is an antagonist at the NMDA receptor and also has actions at adrenergic, muscarinic, seretoninergic and opioid receptors. Its useful actions include potant analgesia, a sympathomimetic effect and a brochodilator action. It is particularly indicated as an induction agent in the shocked or septic patient and the severe asthmatic. Side-effects include hypersalivation, increased intraocular and intracranial pressure and disturbing emergence reactions.

Ref: BJA 1996: 77; 441–444.

2.86 Spironolactone therapy **Answers: B D**

Spironolactone is a potassium sparing diuretic and an antagonist of aldosterone. It thus causes hyperkalaemia and hyponatraemia. The thiazide diuretics cause hyponatraemia, hyperuricaemia, glucose intolerance, hypokalaemia and metabolic alkalosis.

2.87 Intravenous propranolol **Answers: C D**

Propranolol is a non-selective beta-blocking drug. It may cause bronchoconstriction and is both negatively inotropic and chronotropic. In patients receiving verapamil, beta blockers can cause profound hypotension and bradycardia. Although beta blockers mask the response to hypoglycaemia they do not cause hyperglycaemia. Lignocaine is the agent of choice for the treatment of ventricular ectopic beats post myocardial infarction.

2.88 Acute salicylate poisoning **Answers: All false**

Salicylate poisoning commonly causes a respiratory alkalosis and/or a metabolic acidosis. Sweating and hyperpyrexia may occur. Although salicylates may cause gastric irritation and even bleeding it is rarely massive.

2.89 Megaloblastic anaemia **Answers: B C D E**

Megaloblastic anaemia may be caused by deficiency of vitamin B12 or folic acid. The red cells of the blood are macrocytic with an elevated mean corpuscular volume (MCV). Vitamin B12 deficiency is most often due to autoimmune destruction of gastric parietal cells, so called

Addisonian pernicious anaemia (PA). B12 is normally bound by intrinsic factor (IF), produced by gastric parietal cells. The B12 + IF complex is then absorbed in the terminal ileum. Thus disease or surgical resection of stomach or terminal ileum may result in megaloblastic anaemia. As gastric parietal cells produce acid as well as IF achlorhydria is a feature of pernicious anaemia. Gastric cancer is an association of PA. Nitrous oxide can cause megaloblastic anaemia with a normal serum B12. Exposure of > 6 hours can cause this effect by inhibition of the enzyme methionine synthetase. Chronic exposure to nitrous oxide may, rarely, lead to a neurological picture similar to the peripheral neuropathy and sub-acute combined degeneration of the cord seen in vitamin B12 deficiency. Megaloblastosis may be caused by dietary deficiency of folic acid or may be due to anti-folate drugs such as trimethoprim, phenytoin or methotrexate. Other causes of macrocytosis include hypothyroidism, alcohol and liver disease.

2.90 Prothrombin time **Answer: D**

The prothrombin time is a test of the extrinsic pathway of the clotting cascade and is therefore affected by changes in factor 7 or the common pathway. Haemophilia leads to a prolongation of the APTT, as does von Willebrand's disease. In addition the bleeding time is prolonged in von Willebrand's disease. Scurvy, deficiency of vitamin C, leads to defective collagen synthesis. The weak collagen in the vascular connective tissue leads to a prolonged bleeding time. In jaundiced patients there is a deficiency of the vitamin K dependent clotting factors (2, 7, 9 and 10) leading to a prolongation of both the PT and APTT. Thrombocytopenic purpura is due to immune destruction of platelets and only the bleeding time is prolonged.

Viva 1

Examiner 1

Summarise this case.
This is a previously fit woman in the third trimester of her first pregnancy who presents with carpal tunnel syndrome.

What is carpal tunnel syndrome?
Entrapment of the median nerve under the flexor retinaculum at the wrist. The median nerve subserves sensation to the thumb, index, middle fingers; motor to the muscles of the thenar eminence (except adductor policis) and the lateral two lumbricles.

Common causes include pregnancy, rheumatoid arthritis, hypothyroidism, acromegaly and amyloidosis.

Comment on the physical findings and laboratory investigations.
Go through them systematically, explaining why they are normal in the pregnant state.

The murmur is most likely to be a benign flow murmur. Mild oedema is not pathological and that level of proteinuria is not indicative of pre-eclampsia.

How would you anaesthetise this patient?
A regional block is probably the technique of choice. The examiner will expect you to take him through exactly how you would perform, say, a brachial plexus block via the axillary route, including explanation and informed consent from the patient.

Further questions you should anticipate could include:
Comment on the electrophoretic findings. Would this influence your anaesthetic technique?
What local anaesthetic would you use?
What are the effects of a local anaesthetic on the fetus?
If the patient refused a regional block how would you manage this case?
What are the risks to both mother and fetus of general anaesthesia?

Examiner 2

What does this CXR show?
The CXR shows a large pneumothorax of the right lung.

What is your management?
The clinical findings are those of a tension pneumothorax. This is a medical emergency and requires urgent decompression.

1) Oxygen should be given immediately by face mask (as high FiO_2 as possible).
2) An intravenous cannula should be inserted into the right chest immediately.
3) Once stabilised an intercostal drain should be inserted.

(This CXR shows the intercostal drain in situ with re-expansion of the lung.)

Ref.BJHM 1991: 45; 383-386. Management of intercoastal drains.

Tell me about eye blocks for cataract surgery.
The two eye blocks commonly used for cataract surgery are:

1) retrobulbar block
2) peribulbar block

Contraindications to eye block include:

- on anticoagulants/ coagulation problems
- allergy to local anaesthetic drugs
- chronic cough
- inability to lie still or flat

Retrobulbar block:
Local anaesthetic is injected within the muscle cone. Smaller volume of local anaesthetic and faster onset than peribulbar; but greater chance of complications such as retrobulbar haemorrhage (which may cause blindness), injection into CSF, optic nerve damage or penetration of the globe.

Peribulbar block:
Local anaesthetic is injected outside the muscle cone.

Tell me about the problems associated with acute "ecstasy" intoxication
Ecstasy is the street name for the drug 3,4,- methlyenedioxymethamphetamine (MDMA). Taking the drug at "raves" to facilitate prolonged and frenetic dancing may lead to dehydration and a syndrome similar to malignant hyperpyrexia with:

- hyperpyrexia
- muscle rigidity; trismus and bruxism
- rhabdomyolysis
- myoglobinuria and acute renal failure
- disseminated intra vascular coagulation
- multiple organ failure
- obtunded level of consciousness
- seizures

The malignant hyperpyrexia treatment includes:

- rapid cooling measures
- IV dantrolene if temperature is greater than 40 °C
- transfer to ITU
- control seizures
- support failing organ systems
- intubation and ventilation if necessary

Occasionally dancers have consumed vast amounts of water as prophylaxis against dehydration and have then died from water intoxication and the resultant cerebral oedema.

Ref: BJA 1997: 79; 697-8, "Ecstasy" and the Anaesthetist

Viva 2

Examiner 1

Tell me about inotropes.
Inotropes are drugs which increase the force of contraction of cardiac muscle.

Catecholamines increase cAMP and intracellular calcium. They may be endogenous or synthetic.

Adrenaline - beta agonist, some alpha
Noradrenaline - mainly alpha, some beta
Isoprenaline - beta only

Dopamine - alpha, beta and dopamine receptor agonist
Dobutamine - selective beta 1 agonist

- Phosphodiesterase inhibitors
  Specific cardiac phosphodiesterase - Enoximone
  Non-specific phosphodiesterase - aminophylline
  Both increase cAMP by preventing its degradation.

- Cardiac glycosides
  Digoxin alters the ATPase of the Na/K pump.

- Calcium
  Transient effect, increases cytosollic free Ca.

- Glucagon
  Unknown mode of action.

Tell me about the problems of anaesthesia at high altitude.
There is low atmospheric pressure, although FiO2 is the same, the partial pressure is reduced. The need for greater FiO2 makes nitrous oxide a less potent anaesthetic.

Vaporisers
Saturated vapour pressure is unaffected, therefore the partial pressure of the volatile agent is the same. Because atmospheric pressure is reduced the delivered concentration is higher than that shown on the dial. Since anaesthetic action depends on partial pressure, not concentration, the same settings are used as at sea level.

Flowmeters
Since atmospheric pressure is reduced, a given amount of gas occupies a larger volume. Therefore a greater volume of gas is required to pass through the rotameter to maintain a given height. Therefore rotameters under-read. Since it is the number of molecules that is important, the rotameter is used as normal.

Examiner 2

Tell me about postoperative nausea and vomiting.
Causes of postoperative nausea and vomiting include

- Patient factors
  Females
  Young

Anxiety
Travel sickness
Previous PONV
Early mobilization
Eating and drinking

- Anaesthetic factors
  Gastrointestinal distension with gas, hypoxaemia, hypotension
  Drugs - opiates, etomidate, nitrous oxide

- Surgical factors
  Gynaecological surgery
  Ear and eye surgery
  Laparoscopic surgery especially around the stomach

Treatment of postoperative nausea and vomiting includes
- Systematic approach - drugs acting on the periphery (gastrointestinal tract), chemoreceptor trigger zone and the emetic centre
- Antidopaminergic, anticholinergic, antihistaminoid drugs
- The newer anti-5HT3 drugs
- Sympathomimetics

Tell me about the predication of difficult intubation.
There are numerous tests but as the specificity of the tests is poor they will therefore detect many false positives.

- Mallampati Test
  Grades 1-3
  Sensitivity 50%, specificity 96%

- Patil Test
  Thyromental distance 7cm

- Occipito-Atalanto Distance
  A reduction leads to inability to extend the neck at laryngoscopy

- Wilson's Test
  Weight (> 90 kg)
  Head movement
  Jaw protrusion
  Mandibular recession
  Buck teeth
  Score 0-2 for each. A score of > 2 predicts 75% of difficult intubations.

PRACTICE EXAMINATION 3

SHORT ANSWER QUESTION PAPER 3

1. Describe your anaesthetic management of a five-year-old who is bleeding following tonsillectomy 6 hours previously.

2. How would you manage a severely head-injured patient during transfer to a neurological unit?

3. What is your choice of anaesthetic for a primagravid woman at 26/40 gestation requiring appendicectomy?

4. List the possible methods of measuring cardiac output. Describe one method used in intensive care.

5. What are the options for pain relief following a day case circumcision of a two-year-old?

6. What methods of monitoring are available to detect air embolism? Briefly state the problems associated with each method.

7. What are the advantages and disadvantages of the interscalene versus the axillary approaches to the brachial plexus block?

8. Write a letter to be carried by a patient who is thought to be malignant hyperthermia susceptible.

9. Outline the specific complications related to laparoscopic surgery.

10. How may allogeneic blood transfusions be minimised during major surgery?

11. Outline the problems associated with anaesthetising a patient with sickle cell disease for an elective cholecystectomy.

12. How would you pre-operatively assess a patient due for a left pneumonectomy for a bronchogenic carcinoma?

MULTIPLE CHOICE QUESTION PAPER 3

90 Questions: time allowed 3 hours.
Indicate your answers with a tick or cross in the spaces provided.

3.1 Intra-aortic balloon counter pulsation increases

❑ A left ventricular work
❑ B myocardial oxygen requirements
❑ C heart rate
❑ D aortic diastolic pressure
❑ E coronary artery filling

3.2 Recognised complications of bronchial neoplasms include

❑ A hypercalcaemia
❑ B hyperkalaemia
❑ C inappropriate ADH secretion
❑ D Cushing's syndrome
❑ E hypothyroidism

3.3 A laboratory report reading as follows: serum sodium 127 mmol/litre, serum potassium 6.0 mmol/litre, serum chloride 85 mmol/litre, serum bicarbonate 18 mmol/litre, blood urea 18 mmol/litre, fasting blood sugar 3 mmol/litre is compatible with a diagnosis of

❑ A adrenocortical insufficiency
❑ B hepatic failure
❑ C renal failure
❑ D carcinoma of lung with inappropriate antidiuretic hormone secretion
❑ E high small bowel obstruction with vomiting

3.4 A 12-year-old boy is to undergo elective surgery. His older brother died 2 years previously, following an anaesthetic. The parents were told that he died after developing a high fever. Pre-operative investigations should include

- ❑ A a muscle biospy
- ❑ B serum sodium
- ❑ C serum creatine phosphokinase
- ❑ D the fluoride number
- ❑ E plasma cholinesterase level

3.5 A patient develops oliguria after cholecystectomy. The blood urea was 10 mmol/litre preoperatively, and is 33 mmol/l, 2 days after surgery, with a urine osmolality of 300 mOsm/kg and urinary sodium concentration is 140 mmol/l. It is correct to state that

- ❑ A the preoperative blood urea of 10 mmol/l excludes pre-existing renal disease
- ❑ B the urinary sodium concentration would exclude renal disease
- ❑ C the urine osmolality of 300 mOsm/kg water suggests that dehydration and hypovolaemia are the cause of the oliguria
- ❑ D a normal response to stress is suggested by the urinary sodium concentration
- ❑ E the patient is dehydrated

3.6 A patient with central dislocation of the hip following a motor car accident is noted to be shocked on admission, 1 hour after the accident. The most likely causes are

- ❑ A ruptured bladder
- ❑ B blood loss
- ❑ C fat embolism
- ❑ D ruptured urethra
- ❑ E neurogenic shock

3.7 In a patient with head injury the following conditions necessitate surgery:

- ❑ A persistent CSF rhinorrhoea
- ❑ B convulsions
- ❑ C depressed fracture of the skull
- ❑ D extradural haematoma
- ❑ E linear fracture of the skull

3.8 Hypotension associated with the use of methyl methacrylate in total hip replacement is

- ❑ A common after placement of the acetabular prosthesis
- ❑ B associated with entry of the monomer into the blood stream
- ❑ C unrelated to the type of anaesthesia used
- ❑ D aggravated by a high intramedullary pressure
- ❑ E due to pulmonary embolism

3.9 The following features result from acute extracellular depletion of the body fluids:

- ❑ A raised blood urea concentration
- ❑ B raised urine specific gravity
- ❑ C diminished skin elasticity
- ❑ D raised haematocrit
- ❑ E rise in urine osmolality

3.10 The use of large quantities of isotonic non-electrolyte solution for irrigation during prolonged transurethral resection of the prostate may result in

- ❑ A hyponatraemia
- ❑ B haemolysis
- ❑ C haemodilution
- ❑ D hyperkalaemia
- ❑ E hypercalcaemia

3.11 Signs of increasing intracranial pressure after head injury include

- ❑ A a decreasing Glasgow coma score
- ❑ B tachycardia
- ❑ C hypotension
- ❑ D small pupils
- ❑ E an increase in $PaCO_2$

3.12 Obstructive jaundice is associated with

- ❑ A excess urobilinogen in the urine
- ❑ B a palpable gall bladder when due to cholelithiasis
- ❑ C high concentrations of unconjugated bilirubin in the serum
- ❑ D alkaline phosphatase above 100 iu/l
- ❑ E high faecal fat content

3.13 The right main bronchus

- ❑ A lies superior to the right pulmonary artery
- ❑ B is 5 cm long
- ❑ C gives off the upper lobe bronchus before passing posterior to the pulmonary artery
- ❑ D gives off the middle lobe bronchus which then divides into superior and inferior segmental bronchi
- ❑ E is a superior relation of the azygous vein

3.14 Serum creatine phosphokinase activity is characteristically elevated

- ❑ A 24 hours after a myocardial infarction
- ❑ B in osteomalacia
- ❑ C in untreated thyrotoxicosis
- ❑ D in myasthenia gravis
- ❑ E in Duchenne muscular dystrophy

3.15 The following agents may cause pulmonary fibrosis:

- ❑ A bleomycin
- ❑ B cortisone hemisuccinate
- ❑ C beryllium
- ❑ D paraquat
- ❑ E organophosphate compounds

3.16 Carcinoma of the bronchus

- ❑ A may cause dementia
- ❑ B commonly results in a lymphocytic meningitis
- ❑ C may present with a peripheral neuropathy before the primary tumour is demonstrated
- ❑ D may cause cerebellar degeneration without metastasising to the posterior fossa
- ❑ E may cause superior vena caval obstruction

3.17 A patient brought into casualty is found to be gasping for breath and cyanosed. The trachea is deviated to the left and the right side of the chest is hyper-resonant to percussion. He requires

- ❑ A a chest X-ray
- ❑ B an intravenous infusion
- ❑ C immediate needling of the right side of the chest
- ❑ D oxygen given by mask
- ❑ E determination of his acid-base state

3.18 In a patient suffering from chronic respiratory acidosis

- ❑ A there is increased renal excretion of bicarbonate ion
- ❑ B there is an increase in plasma bicarbonate ion concentration
- ❑ C the total buffering ability of the blood is not altered
- ❑ D there is a decrease in the renal excretion of hydrogen ions
- ❑ E there is an equal increase in the number of mmol/l of plasma bicarbonate and carbonic acid

3.19 For the control of postoperative thyrotoxic crisis, the following are indicated at once:

- ❑ A diazepam
- ❑ B digoxin
- ❑ C corticosteroids
- ❑ D propranolol
- ❑ E carbimazole

3.20 After partial gastrectomy the metabolic changes expected in the first 4 days include

- ❑ A hypoglycaemia
- ❑ B a reduction in the amount of sodium excreted in the urine
- ❑ C a decrease in the circulating free fatty acid concentration
- ❑ D an increased excretion of potassium in the urine
- ❑ E an increase in oxygen consumption

3.21 The following may relieve severe pain from osseous metastases of carcinoma of the prostate:

- ❑ A orchidectomy
- ❑ B short wave diathermy
- ❑ C stilboestrol
- ❑ D testosterone
- ❑ E radiotherapy

3.22 The carotid sheath contains the

- ❑ A common carotid artery
- ❑ B vagus nerve
- ❑ C internal jugular vein
- ❑ D sympathetic trunk
- ❑ E ansa hypoglossi nerve

3.23 During one lung anaesthesia hypoxia may be minimised by

- ❑ A hypoxic pulmonary vasoconstriction (HPV)
- ❑ B the application of PEEP to the dependent lung
- ❑ C using large tidal volumes
- ❑ D the application of CPAP to the dependent lung
- ❑ E increasing the inspired oxygen concentration

3.24 Pulse oximeters

- ❑ A can cause burns to the skin under the probe
- ❑ B are inaccurate in the presence of HbF
- ❑ C are inaccurate in the presence of methaemoglobin
- ❑ D are inaccurate in patients with pigmented skin
- ❑ E have a slower response time than transcutaneous oxygen electrodes

3.25 The ECG features of hyperkalaemia include

- ❑ A tall peaked T waves
- ❑ B delta waves
- ❑ C widened QRS complexes
- ❑ D U waves
- ❑ E shortened PR interval

3.26 Paracetamol poisoning

- ❑ A is associated with early metabolic acidosis
- ❑ B is associated with hyperventilation
- ❑ C regularly causes hypothermia
- ❑ D can be treated with acetylcysteine
- ❑ E has been successfully treated with methionine

3.27 Characteristic features of the oliguric stage of acute tubular necrosis include

❑ A the excretion of small amounts of highly concentrated urine
❑ B a progressive rise in central venous pressure
❑ C a high plasma urea with normal creatinine concentration
❑ D malignant hypertension
❑ E hyperkalaemia

3.28 After cardiac arrest

❑ A rapid defibrillation of ventricular fibrillation improves survival dramatically
❑ B calcium is indicated for asystole due to hypokalaemia
❑ C hyperglycaemia should be corrected with insulin
❑ D sodium bicarbonate administration may result in hyperosmolality
❑ E mannitol will reduce cerebral oedema

3.29 Tetanus

❑ A may have an incubation period of over 20 days
❑ B may be prevented by the immediate administration of tetanus toxoid
❑ C may produce severe autonomic disturbances
❑ D should be treated with human antitetanus antitoxin
❑ E is more common with facial wounds than with wounds of the extremities

3.30 Inhalation of 10% oxygen in nitrogen by a normal subject at rest causes

❑ A central cyanosis
❑ B increased cardiac output
❑ C reduction in stroke volume
❑ D a fall in mixed venous oxygen content
❑ E anginal pain

3.31 With refence to colloids

- ❑ A 4.5% albumin has an oncotic pressure similar to blood
- ❑ B hetastarch can prolong the prothrombin time
- ❑ C polygeline can cause acute renal failure
- ❑ D dextran 70 alters red cell deformability
- ❑ E cryoprecipitate is rich in factor VIII

3.32 Ritodrine

- ❑ A slows the heart rate
- ❑ B produces heart block
- ❑ C may cause pulmonary oedema
- ❑ D increases the force of uterine contractions
- ❑ E produces peripheral vasoconstriction

3.33 The following drugs may precipitate bronchospasm:

- ❑ A aspirin
- ❑ B morphine
- ❑ C labetalol
- ❑ D ketamine
- ❑ E isoflurane

3.34 The Wright respirometer tends to underestimate gas volumes when

- ❑ A nitrous oxide is being used
- ❑ B the respirometer is connected directly to the catheter mount
- ❑ C the oxygen contentration is greater than 30%
- ❑ D the tidal volume is low
- ❑ E the vanes are wet

3.35 The meniscus level of a central venous manometer

❑ A is a guide to right ventricular preload
❑ B rises during the inspiratory phase of artificial ventilation
❑ C gives the most accurate readings when the catheter tip lies within the right atrium
❑ D should be measured against a previous base-line zero
❑ E will demonstrate a, c and v oscillations of the central venous pulse if the catheter tip lies within the axillary vein

3.36 Ionised calcium

❑ A should be measured in a sodium heparin (blood gas) sample
❑ B may be measured in a 'clotted' (serum) sample
❑ C is affected by pH
❑ D falls during massive blood transfusion
❑ E is affected by changes in serum protein

3.37 Drug-induced hyperglycaemia may occur with

❑ A bendrofluazide
❑ B captopril
❑ C the oral contraceptive pill (OCP)
❑ D propanolol
❑ E prednisolone

3.38 The signs of a porphyric crisis following anaesthesia are

❑ A weakness of the extremities
❑ B psychosis
❑ C respiratory insufficiency
❑ D renal colic
❑ E passing dark urine

3.39 Halothane vapour

- ❑ A concentration can be measured by using a refractometer
- ❑ B is less dense than nitrous oxide
- ❑ C will absorb ultraviolet radiation
- ❑ D can be measured by infra-red absorption
- ❑ E can be measured by the changes in the elasticity of silicone rubber

3.40 The following will raise the intraocular pressure in a normal eye:

- ❑ A hypercarbia
- ❑ B acetazolamide
- ❑ C atropine
- ❑ D hypotension
- ❑ E respiratory obstruction

3.41 Perioperative hyperkalaemia can follow

- ❑ A intravenous suxamethonium
- ❑ B blood transfusion
- ❑ C intravenous calcium gluconate
- ❑ D intravenous sodium bicarbonate
- ❑ E major trauma

3.42 Nimodipine

- ❑ A is a calcium channel blocker
- ❑ B is cardioselective
- ❑ C is a hypotensive agent
- ❑ D is used for cerebral protection
- ❑ E interacts with aminophylline

3.43 Coeliac plexus block

- ❑ A may relieve pain in abdominal malignancy
- ❑ B may result in orthostatic hypotension
- ❑ C may cause impotence
- ❑ D may be used in the management of chronic pancreatitis
- ❑ E causes constriction of the sphincter of Oddi

3.44 Reactions to intravenous dextrans can be reduced by

- ❑ A slow infusion
- ❑ B giving simultaneous antihistamines
- ❑ C giving a test dose
- ❑ D using hapten dextran before infusion
- ❑ E giving it into a large central vein

3.45 The following drugs are absorbed transdermally:

- ❑ A atropine
- ❑ B hyoscine
- ❑ C morphine
- ❑ D fentanyl
- ❑ E paracetamol

3.46 Propofol

- ❑ A is presented in 20% 'intralipid'
- ❑ B may cause green urine
- ❑ C has little effect on cardiovascular function
- ❑ D reduces ventilatory response to carbon dioxide
- ❑ E has no effect on intraocular pressure

3.47 Bupivacaine

- ❑ A is an amide
- ❑ B is highly protein bound
- ❑ C is contraindicated in malignant hyperpyrexia
- ❑ D may cause refractory arrhythmias
- ❑ E is the drug of choice for intravenous regional anaesthetic

3.48 Premature neonates

- ❑ A are prone to develop hypocalcaemia
- ❑ B are sensitive to non-depolarizing relaxants
- ❑ C have reduced insensible water loss
- ❑ D have increased unconjugated bilirubin levels
- ❑ E are prone to develop hypoglycaemia

3.49 In an infant suffering from persistent vomiting

- ❑ A bile in the vomit is compatible with duodenal atresia
- ❑ B the absence of bile in the vomit favours the diagnosis of pyloric stenosis
- ❑ C a plain X-ray of the abdomen is likely to provide diagnostic help
- ❑ D duodenal atresia is more likely if the child has Down's syndrome
- ❑ E rehydration and gastric aspiration should be undertaken before surgery

3.50 Ventricular ectopic beats occurring during anaesthesia may be treated with

- ❑ A lignocaine
- ❑ B verapamil
- ❑ C beta-adrenoceptor blocking agents
- ❑ D digoxin
- ❑ E carotid sinus pressure

3.51 In cardioversion for cardiac arrhythmias

- ❑ A the shock should be delivered on the upstroke of the T wave
- ❑ B general anaesthesia is not necessary if DC conversion with synchronisation is carried out
- ❑ C AC is safer than DC
- ❑ D no pre-operative preparation is needed for elective cases
- ❑ E ventricular fibrillation may result

3.52 Treatment of pulmonary aspiration of liquid gastric contents of pH less than 2.5 should include

- ❑ A bronchoscopy
- ❑ B bronchial lavage
- ❑ C diuretics
- ❑ D artificial ventilation of the lungs
- ❑ E corticosteroids

3.53 Synthetic oxytocin is preferred to ergometrine for intravenous bolus administration because it

- ❑ A causes less nausea and vomiting
- ❑ B is longer acting
- ❑ C is less likely to produce hypertension
- ❑ D causes less fluid retention
- ❑ E causes less tachycardia

3.54 An obstetrician calls urgently for help because a previously undiagnosed twin has been trapped in the uterus following the injection of ergometrine. Under such circumstances the uterus can be relaxed with the aid of

- ❑ A thiopentone
- ❑ B suxamethonium
- ❑ C d-tubocurarine
- ❑ D halothane
- ❑ E salbutamol

3.55 Cardiovascular changes in pregnancy include

❑ A a fall in mean arterial blood pressure in mid-trimester
❑ B an increase in central venous pressure
❑ C an increase in heart rate
❑ D an increase in total red cell volume
❑ E no change in stroke volume

3.56 Concerning anaphylactic reactions

❑ A they are more common when drugs are given orally
❑ B serum mast cell tryptase is a sensitive diagnostic test
❑ C they are due to degranulation of neutrophils
❑ D isoflurane may relieve refractory bronchospasm
❑ E antihistamines may reduce the severity of a reaction if given before induction of anaesthesia

3.57 Complications of supraclavicular brachial plexus block include

❑ A Horner's syndrome
❑ B phrenic nerve paralysis
❑ C recurrent laryngeal nerve paralysis
❑ D subclavian artery puncture
❑ E accidental subarachnoid injection of local anaesthetic solution

3.58 In axillary brachial plexus block

❑ A the lateral cutaneous nerve of the forearm may be unaffected
❑ B the phrenic nerve may be damaged
❑ C there is a risk of pneumothorax
❑ D Horner's syndrome may occur
❑ E the shoulder muscles may be paralysed

3.59 Concerning intercostal block at the posterior angle of the ribs

- ❑ A the local anaesthetic will spread to segments above and below the site of injection
- ❑ B bilateral blocks should not be performed
- ❑ C the local anaesthetic should be injected between the internal and the innermost intercostal muscles
- ❑ D sympathetic blockade is a recognised complication
- ❑ E addition of adrenaline is contraindicated

3.60 Concerning caudal anaesthesia

- ❑ A there is no risk of dural puncture
- ❑ B the fetal head may be punctured when performed in labour
- ❑ C the volume of local anaesthetic required to block one segment is the same as that required in the lumbar region
- ❑ D a catheter technique cannot be used
- ❑ E the failure rate is higher than for lumbar epidural block

3.61 Epidural test doses are used to

- ❑ A speed onset of analgesia
- ❑ B detect subarachnoid injection
- ❑ C prevent neurological complications
- ❑ D prevent tachyphylaxis
- ❑ E detect intravenous injection

3.62 Ecstasy intoxication

- ❑ A leads to sympathetic overactivity
- ❑ B may be treated with dantrolene
- ❑ C is associated with renal failure
- ❑ D may produce Parkinsonism
- ❑ E may simulate eclampsia if it presents in pregnancy

3.63 Concerning pacemakers and anaesthesia

- ❑ A induction of anaesthesia may alter pacemaker function
- ❑ B unipolar diathermy should be used
- ❑ C a patient with a pacemaker may safely enter an MRI scanner
- ❑ D post-operative shivering may affect pacemaker function.
- ❑ E a magnet placed over a demand pacemaker will convert it to a fixed rate pacemaker

3.64 Concerning Moffet's solution

- ❑ A it contains cocaine at a concentration of 100 mg/ml
- ❑ B it contains adrenaline at a concentration of 0.1 mg/ml
- ❑ C it may lead to ventricular fibrillation in occasional patients
- ❑ D the safe maximum dose for cocaine to the nasal mucosa is 15 mg/kg
- ❑ E it is used to improve post-operative analgesia

3.65 Transplantation of the ureter into the colon may result in

- ❑ A hypochloraemia
- ❑ B a reversible rise in the blood urea
- ❑ C hyperkalaemia
- ❑ D acidosis
- ❑ E hypoglycaemia

3.66 The following may occur in hypothermia:

- ❑ A a delta wave in the ECG
- ❑ B a metabolic acidosis
- ❑ C hypoglycaemia
- ❑ D a raised serum amylase
- ❑ E anaemia

3.67 Dopamine

- ❑ A is a positive inotrope
- ❑ B can be given via a peripheral line
- ❑ C causes tachycardia
- ❑ D stimulates alpha and beta adrenergic receptors
- ❑ E crosses the blood-brain barrier

3.68 Clonidine

- ❑ A is a antisialogogue
- ❑ B may be administered epidurally
- ❑ C causes bradycardia
- ❑ D abrupt withdrawal following chronic administration may cause rebound hypertension
- ❑ E increases the minimum alveolar concentration of the volatile agents

3.69 A post-partum headache may be caused by

- ❑ A post dural puncture headache
- ❑ B subarachnoid haemorrhage
- ❑ C cephalgia fugax
- ❑ D cortical vein thrombosis
- ❑ E herpes simplex encephalitis

3.70 Concerning a Bier's block

- ❑ A 0.5% bupivacaine should be used
- ❑ B the tourniquet may be deflated safely after 10 minutes
- ❑ C the tourniquet should be inflated to 100 mmHg above systolic blood pressure
- ❑ D prilocaine may cause carboxyhaemoglobinaemia
- ❑ E a double tourniquet must be used

3.71 Possible complications of a caudal epidural block include

- ❑ A motor blockade
- ❑ B delayed micturition
- ❑ C subarachnoid block
- ❑ D infection
- ❑ E cauda equina syndrome

3.72 In carbon monoxide poisoning

- ❑ A the pulse oximeter underestimates the oxygen saturation
- ❑ B the oxygen/haemoglobin dissociation curve is shifted to the left
- ❑ C there is histotoxic hypoxia
- ❑ D the arterial oxygen tension is normal
- ❑ E the oxygen content of the blood is normal

3.73 Infantile pyloric stenosis is associated with

- ❑ A hypokalaemia
- ❑ B hyperchloraemia
- ❑ C metabolic acidosis
- ❑ D jaundice
- ❑ E polyuria

3.74 Complex regional pain syndrome type 1 (Reflex sympathetic dystrophy)

- ❑ A may be treated with guanethidine blocks
- ❑ B is associated with allodynia
- ❑ C is associated with hyperalgesia
- ❑ D is associated with osteoporosis of the affected limb
- ❑ E causes purely sensory dysfunction

3.75 In the Report on Confidential Enquiries into Maternal Deaths in the United Kingdom 1991–93

- ❑ A maternal mortality was 1 in 10,000
- ❑ B haemorrhage was the commonest cause of death
- ❑ C the percentage of deaths due to anaesthesia increased from the previous report
- ❑ D there were two fatal anaphylactic reactions to suxamethonium
- ❑ E most deaths due to anaesthesia were due to airway problems

3.76 The measurement of oxygen in a mixture of gases may be made by

- ❑ A pulse oximetry
- ❑ B the Severinghaus electrode
- ❑ C a transcutaneous oxygen electrode
- ❑ D an infrared analyser
- ❑ E mass spectrometry

3.77 Intrathecal narcotics

- ❑ A may cause urinary retention
- ❑ B may cause piloerection
- ❑ C may produce total spinal blockade
- ❑ D may produce pruritus, relieved by propofol
- ❑ E are unlikely to produce significant respiratory depression

3.78 During magnetic resonance scanning

- ❑ A pacemakers are unlikely to malfunction
- ❑ B sudden asphyxia may result due to a quench
- ❑ C ferromagnetic objects may injure the patient
- ❑ D monitoring equipment may be affected by the magnet
- ❑ E objects within the 50 G field may be ferromagnetic

3.79 Unconjugated bilirubin

❑ A is water soluble
❑ B does not cause kernicterus
❑ C is conjugated in the Kupffer cells of the liver
❑ D concentration in the blood in the neonate is influenced by the administration of phenobarbitone to the mother
❑ E is transported in the plasma bound to albumin

3.80 Concerning nitrous oxide

❑ A the cylinder pressure is 137 bar
❑ B the filling ratio is 0.67
❑ C the cylinder pressure falls linearly with use
❑ D the critical temperature is -8 °C
❑ E it can cause vitamin B12 deficiency

3.81 Causes of stridor in a child include

❑ A acute laryngotracheobronchitis
❑ B acute epiglottitis
❑ C inhaled foreign body
❑ D tonsillitis
❑ E bronchiolitis

3.82 The minimum alveolar concentration (MAC) of a volatile agent

❑ A decreases with increasing age
❑ B is increased in pregnancy
❑ C is greater in men than in women
❑ D is greater in neonates than in infants of 2 years of age
❑ E is reduced at altitude

3.83 In one lung anaesthesia the oxygen tension in the blood depends on

- ❑ A the inspired oxygen tension
- ❑ B the intraoperative haematocrit
- ❑ C the mixed venous oxygen tension
- ❑ D the amount of blood flow to the unventilated lung
- ❑ E the cardiac output

3.84 Concerning the Mapleson classification of breathing systems

- ❑ A the Bain system is a Mapleson D system
- ❑ B the Mapleson A system is the most efficient for spontaneous ventilation
- ❑ C there are no valves in the Mapleson E breathing system
- ❑ D all the systems are partial rebreathing systems
- ❑ E the Bain system may be used with some ventilators

3.85 An elderly man arrives in A&E. He is unrousable with a GCS of 6. Blood gases show pH 7.05, PaO_2 8 kPa, $PaCO_2$ 3.2 kPa, bicarbonate 10 mmol/l, Na 135 mmol/l, K 4 mmol/l, urea 6, Cl 95 and glucose 8

- ❑ A he may have taken an overdose of aspirin
- ❑ B he may have taken a methanol overdose
- ❑ C he requires intubation and artificial ventilation
- ❑ D this may be a case of diabetic ketoacidosis
- ❑ E the anion gap is increased

3.86 In Addison's disease

- ❑ A treatment should be with ACTH
- ❑ B the serum sodium is high
- ❑ C there is an inability to excrete a water load
- ❑ D there is hypertension
- ❑ E there is a metabolic alkalosis

3.87 Concerning neonatal physiology

- ❑ A the stroke volume is relatively fixed
- ❑ B low levels of vitamin K dependent clotting factors may cause haemorrhagic disease of the newborn
- ❑ C oxygen consumption is the same as in an adult
- ❑ D they are obligate nasal breathers
- ❑ E circulating blood volume is about 70 ml/kg

3.88 In a patient taking 10 mg of prednisolone daily for rheumatoid arthritis

- ❑ A the steroid should be omitted on the day of operation
- ❑ B excessive doses of glucocorticosteroids increase susceptibility to infection
- ❑ C glucocorticosteroids are needed for the response to surgical stress
- ❑ D the circulating plasma cortisol concentration is normal by 1–2 days after surgical stress in most patients
- ❑ E supplementary hydrocortisone should be given in the peri-operative period

3.89 The following are an indication for oxygen therapy:

- ❑ A carbon monoxide poisoning
- ❑ B haemorrhagic shock
- ❑ C acute asthma attack
- ❑ D diffusion hypoxia
- ❑ E retrolental fibroplasia

3.90 Regarding acute epiglottitis

- ❑ A the causative organism is usually viral
- ❑ B intravenous access should be secured before induction
- ❑ C extubation is usually possible in 48 hours
- ❑ D it only occurs in children
- ❑ E antibiotics are of no benefit

PRACTICE EXAM 3: THE CLINICAL VIVAS

Viva 1: The Clinical Viva takes place in the morning.

1. You are given a piece of clinical information and you have 10 minutes to study it.
2. You will spend 20 minutes with the first examiner, discussing the clinical care of the patient described and how you would anaesthetise for the case.
3. You will then spend 20 minutes with a second examiner discussing approximately three unrelated clinical scenarios.

Viva 2: The Clinical Science Viva takes place in the afternoon. Two examiners will question you for approximately 15 minutes each. Approximately four topics are covered.

A good way to prepare for the viva is to work with a partner. For this reason we have separated the sample questions in this book from the model answers to allow you to work through the viva session before looking at the answers.

Viva 1

Clinical Scenario
A 70-year-old lady presents for open reduction and internal fixation of a fractured tibia and fibula. She suffers with severe rheumatoid arthritis and in addition reflux oesophagitis. She wears a soft neck collar. She has had previous general anaesthetics uneventfully.

Her regular medications are methotrexate, diclofenac and omeprazole. Clinical examination reveals severe rheumatoid hands but is otherwise unremarkable.

Investigations

Hb	8.9 g/dl	Na	140
MCV	69 fl	K	4.5
White count and platelets	Normal	Urea	6.5
		Creatinine	100

The ECG and chest X-ray are normal.
The photograph is of lateral views of the cervical spine in flexion and extension. The X-rays are given in Figs. 4 and 5.

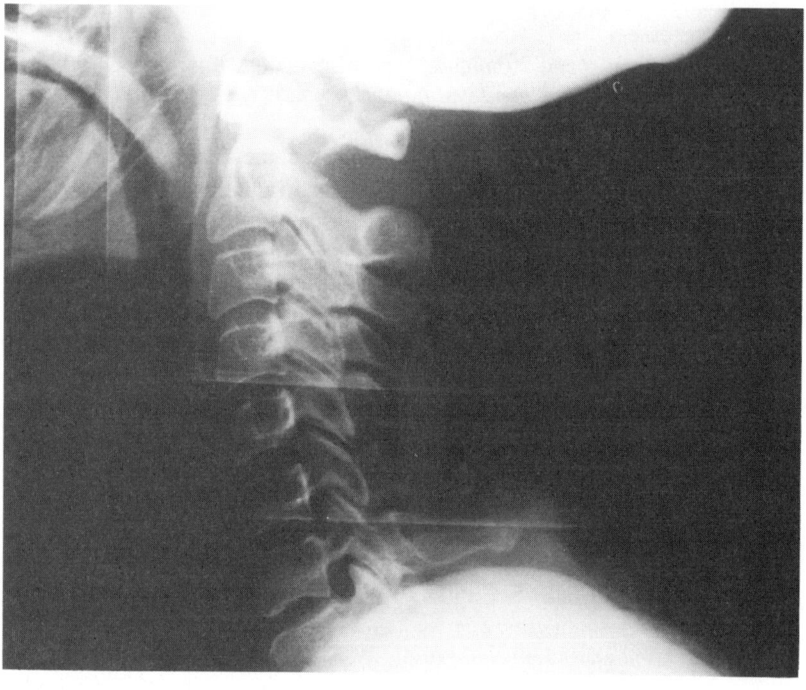

Fig. 4: Cervical spine X-ray

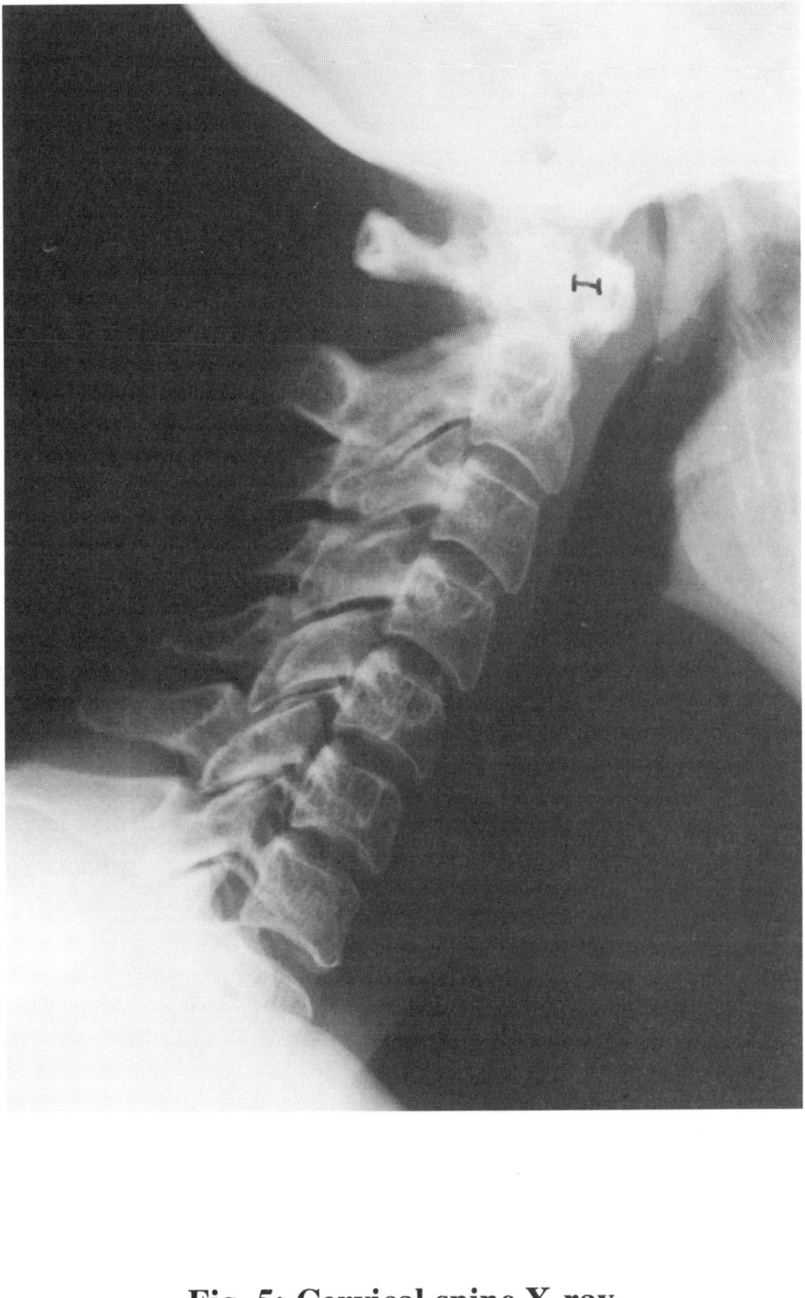

Fig. 5: Cervical spine X-ray

Examiner 1

Summarise the case and the possible and the possible anaesthetic implications.

Describe the findings on the cervical spine X-ray. What is the significance?

How would you anaesthetise this lady?

Examiner 2

Here are a set of arterial blood gases (Table 1) and an ECG (Fig. 6) from a young girl of 16 brought into A&E by her parents having taken some tablets. On arrival she is unconscious with widely dilated pupils. She is tachycardiac and convulsing.

What do you think the diagnosis is?

What is your management?

The second ECG (Fig. 7) was taken 30 mins after her arrival in A&E.

What does it show?

What is your management?

Viva 2

Examiner 1

Here is a PA and lateral chest X-ray (Figs. 8 and 9) of a woman in her 60s presenting for routine orthopaedic surgery. She has never had a previous anaesthetic but takes tablets for weakness.

What does the chest X-ray show?

What is the likely underlying diagnosis?

What is myasthenia gravis?

What medications and other treatments are there for this condition?
What are the anaesthetic implications of myasthenia gravis ?

SYRINGE SAMPLE

ACID/BASE 37°C

pH	6.904↓	
pCO2	7.86↑	kPa
pO2	47.84↑	kPa
HCO3-act	11.4	mmol/L
HCO3-std	9.0	mmol/L
ctCO2	13.2	mmol/L
BE(ecf)	-21.4	mmol/L

OXYGEN STATUS 37°C

ctHb	12.4	g/dL
Hct	36	%
O2CT	8.2	mmol/L
BO2	7.5	mmol/L
pO2	47.84↑	kPa
sO2	98.8↑	%
FO2Hb	96.1	%
FCOHb	1.8↑	%
FMetHb	0.9	%
FHHb	1.2	%

ELECTROLYTES

Na+	144.1	mmol/L
K+	3.29↓	mmol/L
Ca++	1.16	mmol/L
Ca++(7.4)	0.95	mmol/L
Cl-	101	mmol/L
AnGap	35.0	mmol/L

↑ or ↓ = exceeds reference range

Table 1: Arterial blood gases

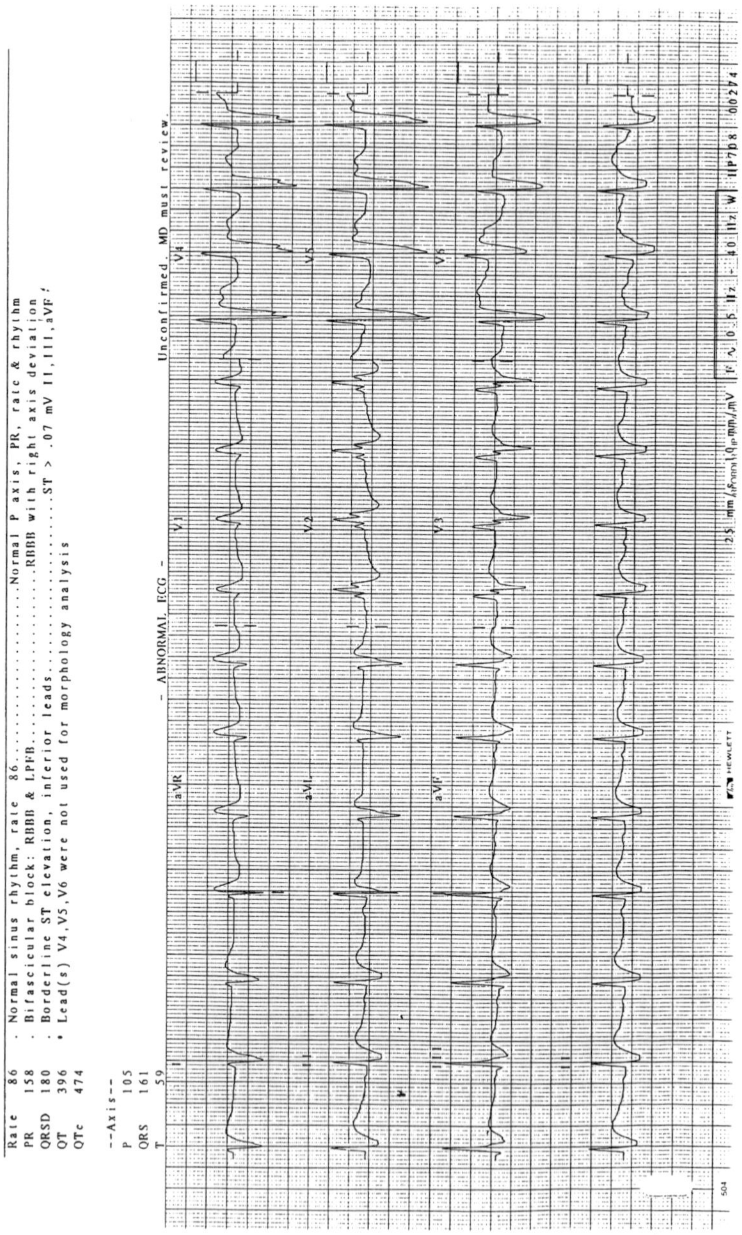

Rate 86 . Normal sinus rhythm, rate 86 ....Normal P axis, PR, rate & rhythm
PR 158 . Bifascicular block: RBBB & LPFB....................RBBB with right axis deviation
QRSD 180 . Borderline ST elevation, inferior leads....................ST > .07 mV II,III,aVF
QT 396 * Lead(s) V4,V5,V6 were not used for morphology analysis
QTc 474
--Axis--
P 105
QRS 161
T 59
- ABNORMAL ECG -
Unconfirmed. MD must review.
I
II
III
aVR
aVL
aVF
V1
V2
V3
V4
V5
V6

Fig. 6: ECG 1

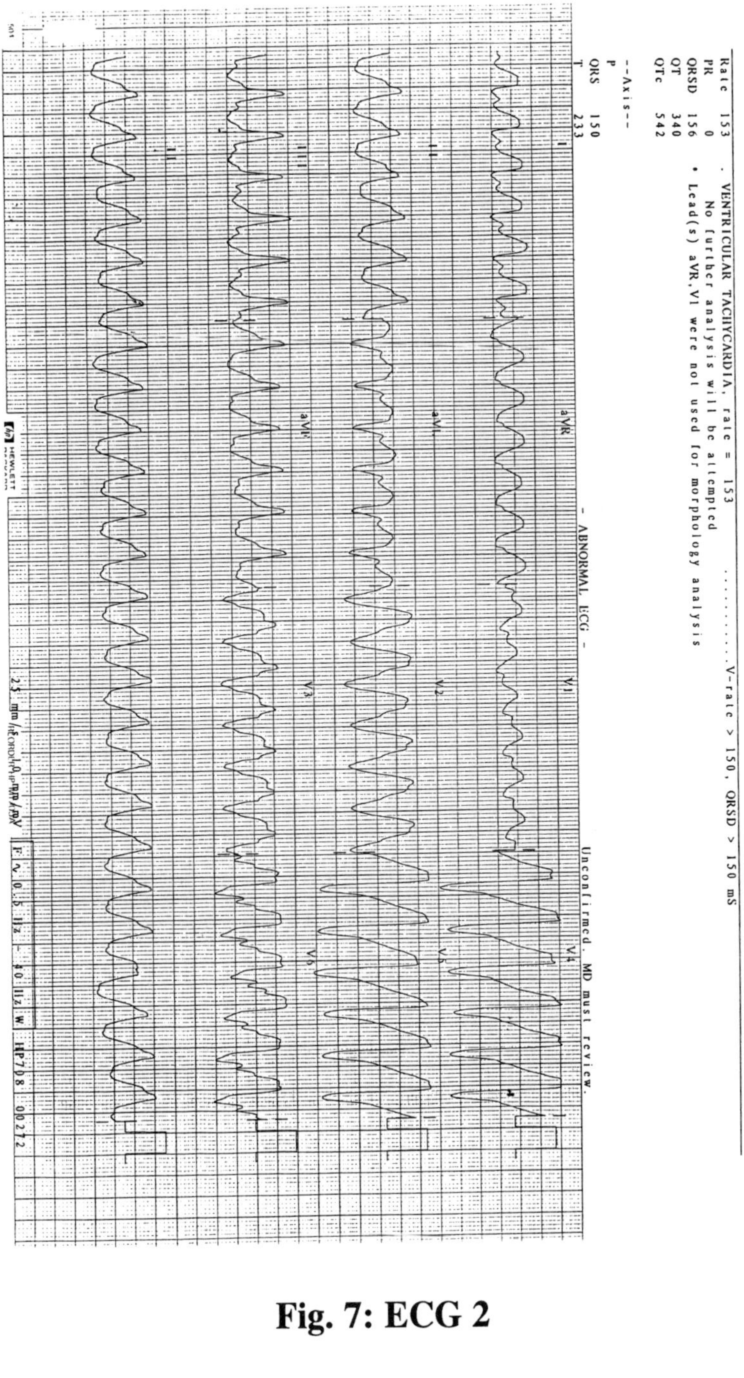
Rate 153
PR 0
QRSD 156
QT 340
QTc 542
--Axis--
P
QRS 150
T 233
. VENTRICULAR TACHYCARDIA, rate = 153 ....V-rate > 150, QRSD > 150 mS
No further analysis will be attempted
• Lead(s) aVR,V1 were not used for morphology analysis
- ABNORMAL ECG -
Unconfirmed. MD must review.
I
II
III
aVR
aVL
aVF
V1
V2
V3
V4
V5
V6

Fig. 7: ECG 2

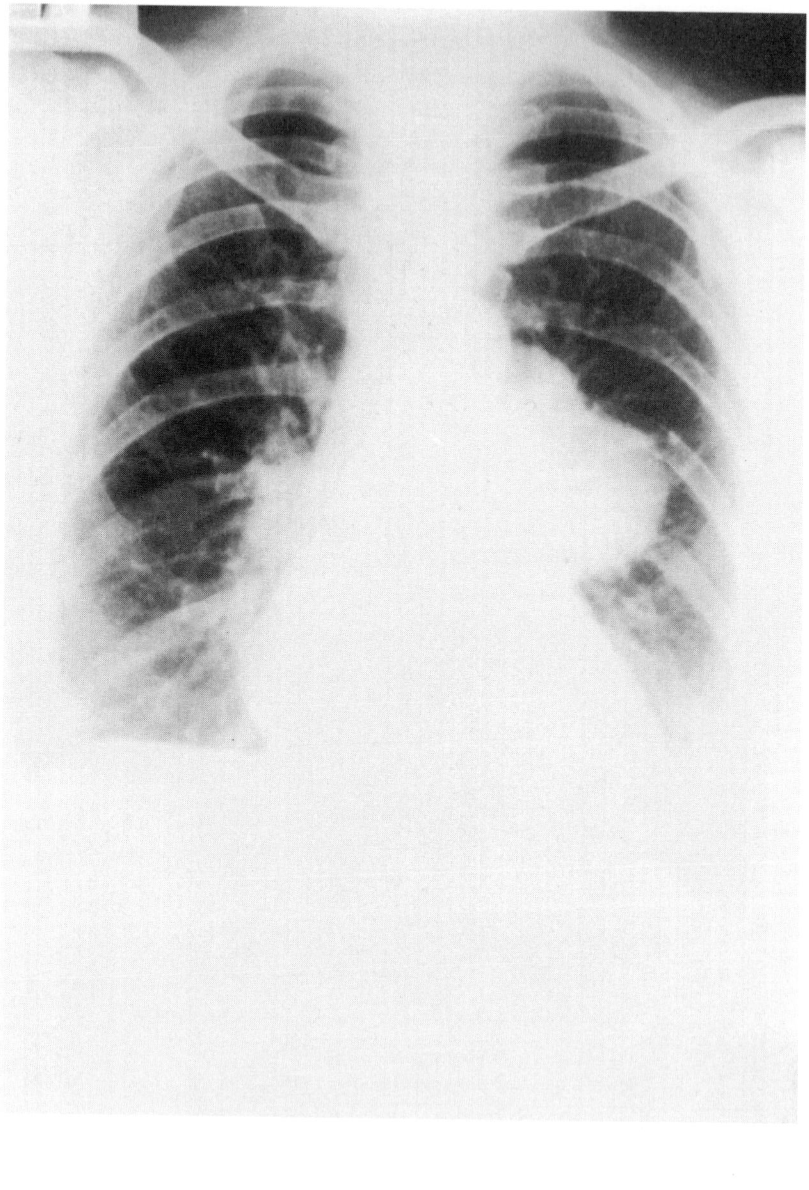

Fig. 8: PA X-ray

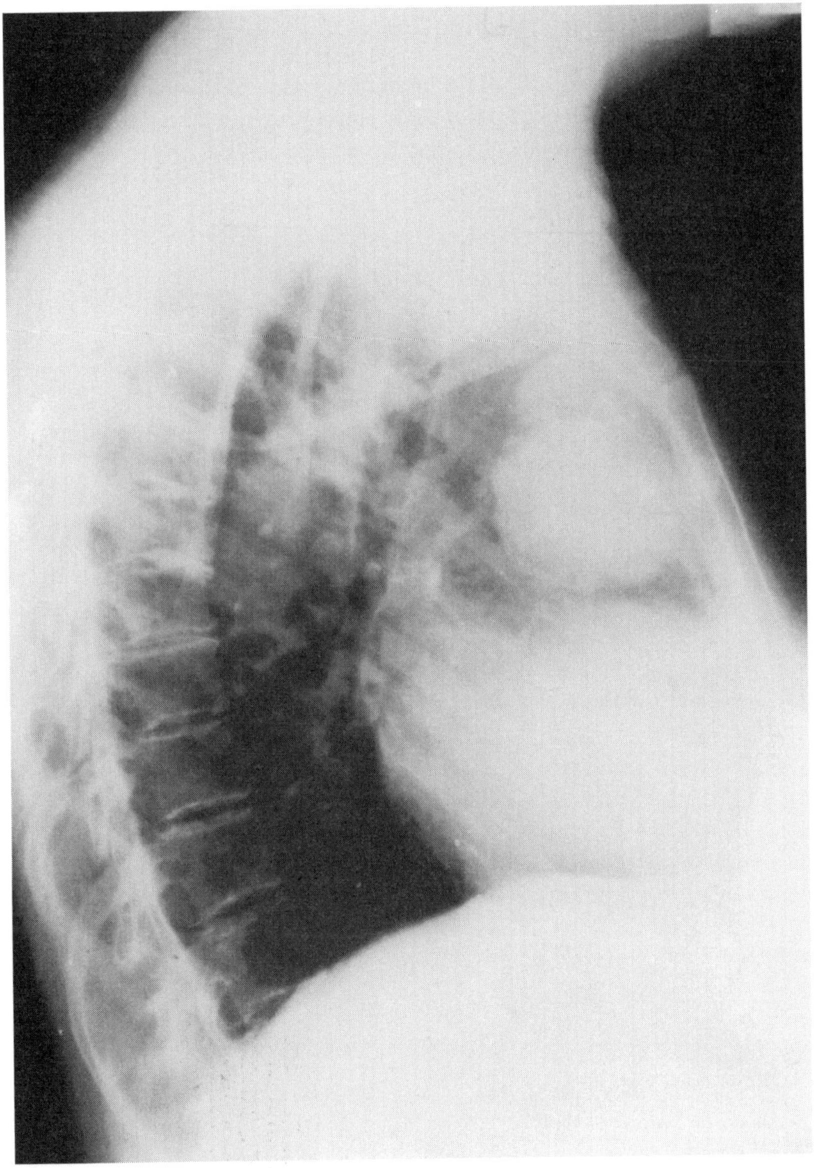

Fig. 9: Lateral X-ray

Examiner 2

Here is a CT scan (Fig. 10) of the brain of a young man who presented to A&E having been knocked unconcious playing rugby. He was initially lucid after regaining conciousness but then lapsed into coma.

What does the scan show?

Describe your initial management of this man in A&E.

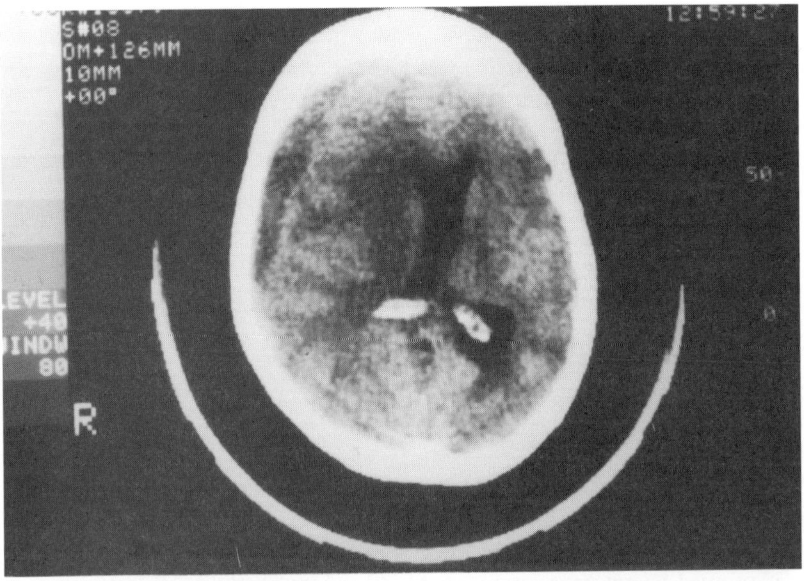

i)

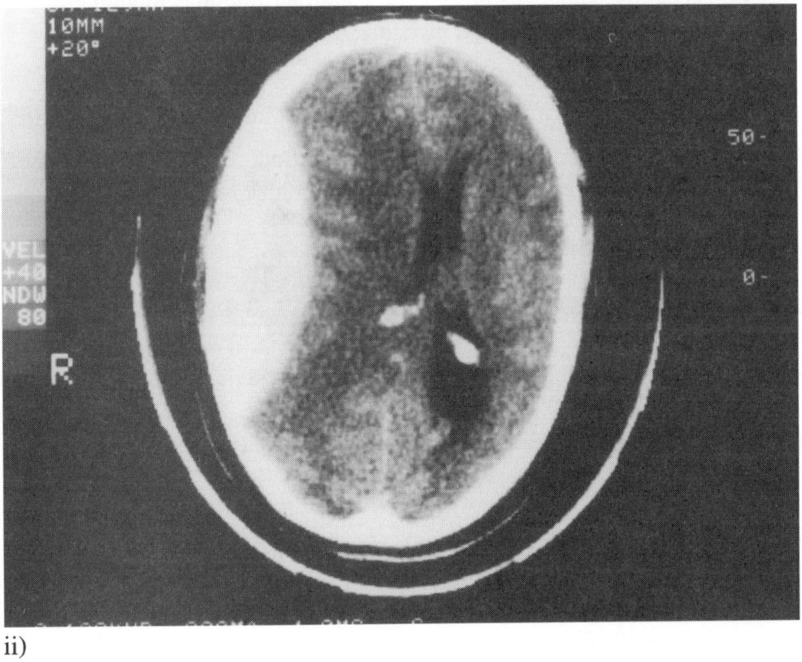

ii)

Fig. 10: CT scans showing i) subdural haematoma and ii) extradural haematoma

SHORT ANSWER QUESTION PAPER 3 ANSWERS

*1. **Describe your anaesthetic management of a five-year-old who is bleeding following tonsillectomy 6 hours previously.***

Problems which must be addressed:

- Haemorrhage – often the amount is underestimated with possible hypovolaemia.
- Swallowed blood and a full stomach predispose to aspiration.
- Potentially difficult airway with blood obscuring the view at laryngoscopy.
- Residual anaesthetic.
- Frightened child and anxious parents.

Preoperative assessment:

- Intravenous access and fluid replacement to ensure normovolaemia with crossmatched blood available.
- Establish whether any anaesthetic difficulties were encountered at the original operation, noting particularly endotracheal tube size.
- Consider emptying the stomach with a nasogastric tube, though this may cause more distress and bleeding; or premedication with atropine and an anti-emetic.

Anaesthetic management:

- Ensure adequate resuscitation prior to induction.
- Full monitoring prior to induction on tilting table head down, with effective suction.
- Rapid sequence induction with cricoid pressure, thiopentone and suxamethonium.
- Endotracheal intubation which may require a smaller sized tube than before.
- Maintenance with nitrous oxide, oxygen and isofurane spontaneously breathing through a T-piece.
- Prior to extubation wash the stomach out via a nasogastric tube.
- Extubate head down on side fully awake.

Postoperatively:

- Check Hb
- Beware of airway obstruction if the throat has been packed or if pre-existing sleep apnoea.
- Consider high dependency unit for close monitoring.

2. ***How would you manage a severely head-injured patient during transfer to a neurological unit?***

Problems to be addressed:

- Potentially unstable patient, transferred in isolated environment with limited equipment and personnel.
- Continuation of therapy to avoid secondary brain injury.
- Prior to transfer it may be indicated to intubate patient (if not already intubated) especially if fluctuating level of consciousness, swelling or bleeding from face injuries may make intubation more difficult or seizures (remember cervical spine control during intubation).
- Associated injuries (present in 30%) sought and managed prior to transfer.
- Adequate resuscitation of any associated injuries.
- Appropriate personnel – at least one trained assistant.
- Equipment appropriate to patient – including ventilator, oxygen and reserve drugs, fluids and blood, as well as alternative method of ventilation (ambu-bag) should ventilator oxygen fail.

Continuation of therapy to avoid secondary brain injury:

- Ensure adequate flux oxygen to brain tissue with impaired autoregulation.
- High inspired oxygen, either by face mask or ventilator.
- Ensure mean arterial pressure adequate to perfuse brain despite rising intracranial pressure – either by use of fluids and or inotropes.
- Aim to limit rising intracranial (this may only be possible by definitive neurosurgical intervention).
- Moderate hyperventilation to $PaCO_2$ 4–4.5 kPa.
- Avoid straining, coughing.
- Avoid tight endotracheal ties, venous congestion.
- Ensure adequate sedation prior to movement or intervention (e.g. suctioning), consider mannitol if acute deterioration (unilateral increase in pupil size).
- Careful continued monitoring including invasive blood pressure, ECG, PaO_2 and $ETCO_2$ together with frequent clinical evaluation – pupil size in paralysed ventilated patient.
- Glasgow coma scale in un-intubated patient.

3. ***What is your choice of anaesthetic for a primagravid woman at 26/40 gestation requiring appendicectomy?***

General considerations:

- Safe anaesthesia for woman, remembering physiological changes of pregnancy.
- Fetal considerations, maintaining placental blood flow, avoidance of teratogens.

Preoperative management:

- Thorough assessment, particularly airway may need rehydration with intravenous fluids.
- Acid aspiration prophylaxis, ranitidine and sodium citrate.
- Liaise with obstetric staff for fetal monitoring pre- and postoperative.
- Avoid aortocaval compression, transportation in left lateral position.
- Graduated compression stockings advisable as hypercoagulability and venous stasis predispose to thromboembolism.
- Rapid sequence induction and intubation with pre-oxygenation, 15 degree tilt and cricoid press using thiopentone and suxamethonium (no anaesthetic drugs have been conclusively proven to be safe or teratogenic).
- Maintenance using IPPV relaxant, oxygen and volatile agent with supplemental opioid.
- Extubation in left lateral position, fully awake, ensure good oxygenation and continue fetal monitoring.
- Analgesia provided by opioids often using patient-controlled analgesia system.
- Avoidance of non-steroidal anti-inflammatories due to the theoretical risk of premature ductus closure in utero.

4. ***List the possible methods of measuring cardiac output. Describe one method used in intensive care.***

Cardiac output: the volume of blood pumped by the heart per minute.

- Fick principle: usually oxygen consumption is measured. Requires samples of arterial and mixed venous blood to calculate their oxygen content.

$$O_2 \text{ consumption} = (CaO_2 - C\bar{v}O_2) \times CO$$

- Dilutional techniques. Either dye or cold saline are used as indicators.
- Transoesophageal echocardiography using the Doppler effect. The velocity of blood in the ascending aorta is measured, when multiplied by the aortic cross-sectional area gives the stroke volume.
- Cardiac catheterization. Highly invasive giving an estimate of stroke volume.
- Radioisotope scanning. Gives an average stroke volume over a long time period. Unsuitable for rapid variations.
- Echocardiography. Two-dimensional view gives an estimate of stroke volume. Large inter operator variability.
- Impedance plethysmography. A research tool.

Dilutional techniques:

- Most commonly used in intensive care. Requires pulmonary artery catheterization.
- Cold saline is used as the indicator for repeated measurements. A thermistor situated at the catheter tip measures the change in temperature.
- 5–10 ml of saline is injected at end expiration into the proximal port (RA) of the pulmonary artery catheter.
- The change in temperature of blood passing through the pulmonary artery is detected against time. A semi-logarithmic plot is made: temperature change against time. The area under the curve gives the cardiac output.
- The average of three measurements is taken.
- Cold water indicator avoids the second peak of dye recirculation and allows repeated measurements in critically ill patients.

5. ***What are the options for pain relief following day case circumcision in a two-year-old?***

- Requirement for adequate analgesia with low incidence of side-effects.
- Variable response of children to opiate analgesics with potential for serious side-effects of sedation and respiratory depression make them less useful in day case setting.
- Non-steroidal drugs are a useful adjunct though insufficient alone. Unsuitable for children with asthma as they may precipitate bronchospasm.
- Regional techniques are popular, providing local analgesia with minimal side-effects.
  Penile block. Dorsal nerves of the penis derive from the pudendal nerve. May be blocked by injection of 2–5 ml of 0.25% plain bupivicaine inferior to the symphysis pubis in the mid line below Buck's fascia. Genital branch of the genitofemoral blocked separately by subcutaneous infiltration on the ventral surface. Good quality analgesia, few side-effects: haematoma, misplacement of solution, urinary retention unlikely.
  Caudal analgesia. 0.5 ml/kg of 0.25% bupivicaine injected through sacrococcygeal membrane. Provides good quality analgesia but frequent side-effects; urinary retention and weakness of lower limbs. Complications include intravascular injection, dural puncture and technical difficulty due to anatomical variation (5%).
- Simple oral analgesia such as paracetamol is usually sufficient following the acute phase.

6. *What methods of monitoring are available to detect air embolism? Briefly state the problems associated with each method.*

Awake patient

- Will complain of chest pain and dyspnoea preceding cardiovascular collapse.

Basic senses and a high index of suspicion

- At risk operations include neurosurgical and orthopaedic. Hissing may be heard over the surgical field. Subjective and insensitive.

Heart sounds

- Millwheel murmur heard using a praecordial stethoscope. Insensitive needing 1.5–4.0 ml of air/kg by which time there may be cardiovascular collapse.

ECG

- Signs of right ventricular strain or arrythmias. Non-specific.

CVP

- An abrupt rise due to outflow obstruction of the right heart. Again non-specific.

Capnography

- Air emboli are trapped in the pulmonary vessels causing a rapid rise in physiological dead space and an abrupt decrease in end tidal carbon dioxide. Able to detect 1.5 ml/kg prior to cardiovascular collapse.

Transthoracic Doppler

- Placed in the 4th right interspace it can detect 0.5 ml of air by change in signal. However, over-sensitivity (0.5 ml of air may be inconsequential), interference from diathermy and difficulty maintaining patient contact limit its use.

Transoesophageal echocardiography

- More sensitive than Doppler but will not differentiate between air, fat or blood microemboli.

7. ***What are the advantages and disadvantages of the interscalene versus the axillary approaches to the brachial plexus block?***

Technical ease:

- Interscalene more difficult landmarks than axillary with its constant relationship to the axillary artery.
- Axillary approach allows indwelling catheter to be inserted for repeated injections.

Clinical application:

- Interscalene reliably blocks structures innervated by C5–C7; the deep tissues of the shoulder, elbow joint and superficial areas of the radial aspect of the forearm. however it inconsistently blocks the lower roots of the plexus.
- Axillary approach consistently blocks the medial aspects of arm, forearm and hand (median and ulnar nerves) however radial and musculocutaneous are blocked in only 75% cases and the circumflex nerve is unreliably blocked.

Complications:

- Those of interscalene are numerous and may be serious compared with axillary.

Interscalene:

- Phrenic nerve block: 36% patients radiographically
- Recurrent laryngeal nerve block, hoarseness
- Horner's syndrome: 50% patients
- Vertebral artery injection, causing severe cerebral toxicity
- Epidural and subarachnoid injection

Axillary:

- Haematoma, especially if transarterial method is used
- Intravascular injection

8. *Write a letter to be carried by a patient who is thought to be malignant hyperthermia susceptible.*

To whom it may concern:
Re: A R Bloggs
DOB: ?/??/??

This patient developed masseter spasm following an appendicectomy and was subsequently investigated for malignant hyperthermia. A biopsy of vastus medialis showed contraction to both caffeine, 2 mmol/l, and halothane 2%. This patient is therefore malignant hyperthermia susceptible.

If general anaesthesia is necessary, a volatile-free anaesthetic machine (produced by flushing a vaporiser free machine with oxygen 8 l/min for 20 minutes) should be used together with a new ventilator and tubing.

Suxamethonium, all volatiles, amide local anaesthetics and sympathetic vasoconstrictors should all be avoided during anaesthesia. Monitoring should include temperature, capnography and oximetry. Dantrolene should be available within the operating theatre.

A national register of MH susceptible individuals is kept in Leeds, from which further information may be obtained.

Yours sincerely

9. ***Outline the specific complications related to laparoscopic surgery.***

Cardiovascular collapse

- Raised intra-abdominal pressure (IAP), reduced venous return and high systemic vascular resistance lead to low cardiac output. Aim to keep the IAP < 15 mmHg and ensure normovolaemia.

Respiratory compromise

- Pneumoperitoneum splints the diaphragm, reduces FRC and compliance and therefore worsens V/Q mismatch. Resulting in hypoxaemia and hypercarbia. This is compounded by peritoneal absorbtion of carbon dioxide leading to acidosis and dysrythmias.

Gas embolism

- Due to insertion of trochar into blood vessel. Carbon dioxide used as insufflating gas is highly soluble to reduce this risk.

Visceral damage

- Due to limited view via the scope it may go unnoticed presenting as peritonitis at a later date.

Haemorrhage

- May be difficult to assess, especially if retroperitoneal.

Hypothermia

- Particularly a problem with long operations and use of cold insufflating gas.

Venous stasis and thromboembolism

- Due to high intra-abdominal pressures obstructing flow in the inguinal veins.

Escape of insufflating gas

- Pneumothorax or pneumoperitoneum may occur if the pleuro-peritoneal canals are patent. Surgical emphysema and shoulder tip pain are common.

Ref: Anaesthesia Review 11. 1996. 13th Edition, Kaufman, CL.

10. How may allogeneic blood transfusions be minimised during major surgery?

Autologous blood transfusion

- Predonation. Requires planning and assistance from haematology department. One unit donated per week, up to six units with iron supplements. Suitable for fit patients only.
- Haemodilution. Whole blood is venesected following induction of anaesthesia and replaced with colloid.
- Blood salvage. For major vascular, hepatic and cardiac surgery. Complicated, expensive equipment. Blood is washed and resuspended in saline, coagulopathy is a problem. Contraindicated in the presence of bacteria or tumour cells.

Limitation of perioperative blood loss

- Tourniquets. Suitable only for limb surgery. Pressure necrosis under the tourniquet and limb ischaemia limit the available time. Unsuitable in sickle cell disease.
- Local infiltration with sympathomimetic amines. Adrenaline 1:200–400 000 is commonly used to cause local vasoconstriction in the surgical field.
- Hypotensive anaesthesia. Controversial. Many contraindications; cerebrovascular disease, ischaemic heart disease, hypertension, diabetes, pregnancy, anaemia. Multiple anaesthetic techniques exist to induce hypotension.

Use of synthetic oxygen-transporting blood substitutes

Presently only in experimental stages. Modified haemoglobin from various sources including recombinant DNA techniques may reduce allogeneic transfusion in future.

Ref: BJA 1992: 69; 489–507.

11. *Outline the problems associated with anaesthetising a patient with sickle cell disease for an elective cholecystectomy.*

- An inherited group of disorders characterized by variable amounts of haemoglobin S. Patients are usually SS but may be SC or S beta thal.
- Haemoglobin S in the deoxygenated form becomes insoluble forming sickle shaped red cells. A process promoted by hypoxia, acidosis, dehydration and low temperature.
- Chronic sickling leads to reduced microvascular blood flow (and end organ damage) and chronic haemolytic anaemia (Hb 6–10 g/dl) with frequent gall stones.

Problems:

Evaluation of pre-existing end organ damage

- Cardiomegaly or cardiomyopathy. Raised cardiac output due to anaemia.
- Occult pulmonary infarction, possible pulmonary hypertension.
- Renal medullary infarction with impaired renal function and concentrating ability.

Prevention of peri-operative sickle crisis:

- Consultation with a haematologist. Exchange transfusion over 6–8 weeks pre-operatively may be indicated aiming for Hb > 8 g/dl and HbA > 40%.
- Pre, per and post operative hypoxia, acidosis, hypothermia and dehydration are avoided.
- Sedative premedication is avoided. Intravenous hydration from the time of starvation.
- Pre-oxygenation with a smooth anaesthetic induction, intubation and moderate hyperventilation.
- Adequate warmed fluid replacement to maintain cardiac output and prevent vascular sludging.
- Careful intra-operative monitoring including pulse oximetry, urine output and temperature with use of active warming measures if necessary.
- Postoperative HDU care to ensure adequate analgesia, avoidance of hypoxia, dehydration or hypotension.

Increased risk of infection

- Auto splenectomy places patients at increased risk, prophylactic antibiotics are advisable.

12. How would you pre-operatively assess a patient due for a left pneumonectomy for a bronchogenic carcinoma?

General assessment

Pre-operative assessment including history, examination and investigation. Patients tend to be elderly, present or past smokers with concurrent cardio-respiratory disease.

Assessment of cardio-respiratory function

- Clinical examination to detect dyspnoea at rest or on exertion, sputum production and purulence, signs of right ventricular failure or bronchospasm.
- ECG to detect signs of RV strain or ischaemic heart disease.
- CXR and ABGs to document baseline values.
- Full blood count and electrolytes.
- CT scan of the chest may indicate any tracheal deviation or large airway collapse.
- Lung function tests. These will also be useful in predicting the risk of pneumonectomy. Peak expiratory flow rate (PEFR) spirometry to produce FEV1 and FVC and any response to bronchodilators.

Assessment of any paraneoplastic syndrome

- Bronchial carcinomas frequently produce hormone-like substances. Resulting biochemical abnormalities may need correction pre-operatively.
- Hypercalcaemia from PTH-like substance.
- Inappropriate ADH.
- Cushing's syndrome.
- Eaton-Lambert syndrome: non-fatiguable weakness of skeletal muscle.

Evaluation of the risk of pneumonectomy

- Left pneumonectomy comprises 40% of lung function. However pre-operative lung function may reflect a functional pneumonectomy if the lesion is occluding the main bronchus.
- No clear cut criteria exist for selection of patients who will tolerate a pneumonectomy.

  However FEV1 > 0.8l is needed for an adequate cough.
  FEV1 < 1.0l patients may have difficulty clearing secretions.

  Maximal breathing capacity (MBC) < 35 correlates with poor outcome
  MBC = PEFR x 0.25

  Postoperative pulmonary hypertension is a significant cause of mortality. Efforts are now made to mimic the postoperative situation using pulmonary artery catheters. Mean PA pressures > 40 mmHg are indicative of poor outcome.

MCQ PAPER 3 ANSWERS

3.1 Intra-aortic balloon **Answers: D E**

The intra-aortic balloon pump (IABP) is inserted via the femoral artery and positioned in the descending aorta, just distal to the left subclavian artery. Inflation is synchronised to the patient's ECG. It is inflated with 50 ml of helium or carbon dioxide at the onset of diastole.This results in displacement of blood into the proximal and distal aorta, increasing aortic diastolic pressure. This in turn leads to improved coronary artery perfusion and increased myocardial oxygen delivery. It is deflated just prior to systole so decreasing left ventricular afterload, left ventricular work and myocardial oxygen requirements.

Ref: BMJ 1993: 307; 35–41.

3.2 Bronchial neoplasms **Answers: A C D**

Bronchial carcinomas may produce a variety of ectopic hormones such as ACTH, causing Cushing's syndrome with hypokalaemia and parathormone causing hypercalcaemia. The syndrome of inappropriate production of antidiuretic hormone (SIADH) may occur. Hypercalcaemia can also occur if there are bony secondaries.

3.3 Syndrome of inappropriate anti-diuretic hormone **Answer: A**

SIADH leads to retention of water and both the serum sodium and potassium are reduced. Bowel obstruction with vomiting leads to hypokalaemia. In hepatic failure the urea is low as the liver fails to synthesise it. In renal failure the serum sodium is normal and there is no hypoglycaemia. Addison's disease fits the metabolic picture precisely. Lack of cortisol leads to loss of sodium chloride and retention of potassium, as well as hypoglycaemia. The urea is elevated and there is a metabolic acidosis.

3.4 Malignant hyperpyrexia **Answers: A C**

The history points to a diagnosis of malignant hyperpyrexia as the cause of death in the patient's brother. The serum creatine phosphokinase is a useful marker for this condition but lacks both specificity and sensitivity. A muscle biopsy is required so that the in vitro contracture tests can be performed. This involves exposing muscle to halothane and caffeine. The fluoride number and plasma cholinesterase level are tests for the presence of atypical plasma cholinesterase, so called scolene apnoea.

3.5 Oliguria **Answers: All false**

The pre-operative blood urea of 10 mmol/l suggests existing renal disease. Postoperatively the patient's urea rises further and small amounts of poor quality urine are produced. The normal response to stress involves release of ADH and aldosterone leading to retention of sodium and water.

3.6 Neurogenic shock **Answer: B**

Neurogenic shock implies a significant head injury; there is nothing in the history to suggest this. A ruptured urethra would not cause shock. Fat embolism usually occurs later than 1 hour after the accident and causes hypoxia and confusion. Shock is not a major feature. Blood loss is the likeliest explanation for the clinical findings.

3.7 Head injury **Answers: A C D**

A extradural haematoma following a head injury is due to bleeding from the middle meningeal artery. It requires surgical evacuation. Persistent CSF rhinorrhoea and a depressed skull fracture will also require surgery, but a linear fracture does not. Convulsions require treatment with anticonvulsants but do not necessarily indicate that the patient requires surgery.

3.8 Methyl methacrylate in total hip replacement **Answers: A D E**

The cement implantation syndrome is characterised by systemic hypotension, pulmonary hypertension and oxygen desaturation at the time of cement and prosthesis insertion. It is now thought to be caused by the haemodynamic effects of emboli and not by the toxic properties of methyl methacrylate monomer. Embolisation results from high intramedullary pressures. The underlying problem is acute pulmonary hypertension and secondary right ventricular failure. This causes a decrease in left ventricular function and a reduction in cardiac output. Coronary perfusion pressure is decreased by the hypotension and may lead to ischaemia and infarction in patients with coronary artery disease. Anaesthetic factors may influence the cardiovascular response to the surgically-induced embolic load. Intravascular volume depletion will aggravate the severity of the hypotension and the volatile agents may predispose to more pronounced haemodynamic effects for a given embolic load.

Ref: Canadian J Anaesthetics 1997: 44; 107–111.

3.9 Extracellular depletion of body fluids **Answers: A B C D E**

In response to acute extracellular depletion of body fluids the kidneys produce renin and the pituitary produces ADH. There is a rise in blood urea and haemoconcentration. Renin leads to increased aldosterone release from the adrenal cortex which in turn leads to retention of sodium. The ADH leads to water retention. The result is the production of small amounts of concentrated urine.

3.10 TUR syndrome **Answers: A C**

The TUR syndrome results from the absorption of large amounts of irrigating fluid into the vascular space. The biochemical effects are due to haemodilution and include hyponatraemia, hypokalaemia and hypocalcaemia. Irrigating fluid is isotonic and so does not cause haemolysis.

3.11 Increasing intracranial pressure **Answers: A E**

Increasing intracranial pressure leads to a decline in the Glasgow coma score. In addition there is usually hypertension with reflex bradycardia. The hypertension is an attempt to maintain cerebral perfusion pressure as: cerebral perfusion pressure = mean arterial pressure – intracranial pressure. The pupils are dilated and respiratory depression leads to an increase in $PaCO_2$.

3.12 Obstructive jaundice **Answer: E**

Obstructive jaundice is most commonly due to either pancreatic carcinoma or gallstones. The hallmark of obstructive jaundice is pale stools and dark urine. The stools are pale due to a lack of faecal stercobilinogen. Bilirubin causes the dark urine. Since liver function is normal (only excretion of the bile is impeded) the bile is thus normally conjugated. The liver enzymes alkaline phosphatase and gamma glutamyl transpeptidase are disproportionately elevated with respect to the transaminases. The alkaline phosphatase is often well in excess of 1000 iu/l, the normal range being 30–300 iu/l. With gallstones the gallbladder is usually fibrotic and shrunken. A palpable gallbladder suggests pancreatic carcinoma (Courvoisier's sign). In obstructive jaundice there may be a high faecal fat content since bile salts are necessary for fat absorption from the gut. The fat-soluble vitamins, such as vitamin K, are not absorbed either. Lack of vitamin K prevents hepatic synthesis of the clotting factors 2, 7, 9 and 10 resulting in prolongation of the PT and APTT.

obstructive jaundice γGT & ALK ↑ > ALT, AST

3.13 Right main bronchus **Answers: A C**

The right main bronchus, after 2.5 cm, gives off the right upper lobe bronchus, which in turn trifurcates to give the apical, anterior and posterior segments. The right main bronchus continues a further 2 cm before giving off the middle lobe bronchus, which in turn bifurcates into the lateral and medial segments of the right middle lobe.The right main bronchus, at 4.5 cm, is slightly shorter than the left which is 5 cm in length. The right main bronchus lies superior and posterior to the right pulmonary artery and inferior to the azygous vein.

3.14 Serum creatine phosphokinase **Answers: A E**

The enzyme creatine kinase (CK) has three iso-enzymes:

1) CK-BB found in brain tissue
2) CK-MM found in muscle tissue
3) CK-MB found in myocardial tissue

An elevated creatine kinase can be seen 24 hours after a myocardial infarct, in Duchenne muscular dystrophy and in hypothyroidism. Osteomalacia leads to an increase in the enzyme alkaline phosphatase, which can be produced by osteoblasts or hepatocytes; hence it is elevated in liver disease as well.

3.15 Pulmonary fibrosis **Answers: A C D**

The causes of pulmonary fibrosis are legion but include paraquat, bleomycin and beryllium. Other drugs that may cause pulmonary fibrosis include amiodarone, cyclophosphamide and nitrofurantoin. Occupational exposure to silicates and asbestos may cause fibrosis of the lungs.

3.16 Carcinoma of the bronchus **Answers: A C D E**

Carcinoma of the bronchus is associated with a number of non-metastatic extrathoracic complications. These include the Eaton-Lambert myaesthenic syndrome, peripheral neuropathy, cerebellar degeneration and dementia. The tumour can cause superior vena caval obstruction and may, rarely, cause a lymphocytic meningitis.

3.17 Tension pneumothorax **Answers: C D**

The clinical findings are those of a tension pneumothorax, which is a medical emergency. The patient requires oxygen and immediate needling of the right side of the chest. Once stabilised a chest drain with underwater seal can be inserted until the right lung has completely re-expanded.

3.18 Chronic respiratory acidosis **Answer: B**

Chronic respiratory acidosis is due to carbon dioxide retention, as occurs in chronic bronchitis. To restore pH towards normal the kidneys retain bicarbonate ions and excrete hydrogen ions.

3.19 Postoperative thyrotoxic crisis **Answers: A D**

To control the tachycardia and agitation of post-operative thyrotoxic crisis diazepam and propranolol should be given at once. Carbimazole will not work immediately and should be given once the initial situation is controlled.

3.20 Major surgery **Answers: B D E**

After major surgery the body produces increased amounts of renin, ADH and cortisol leading to hyperglycaemia and renal retention of sodium and water and excretion of potassium. The patient is in a catabolic state and there is increased excretion of nitrogen and increased consumption of oxygen. Muscle and adipose tissue are broken down to supply energy leading to an increased level of circulating free fatty acids.

It is thought that many of these metabolic responses are mediated by cytokines, especially interleukin-1, interleukin-6 and tumour necrosis factor-alpha. The rise in IL-6 is a good measure of the degree of tissue injury, and there is evidence that anaesthesia can attenuate the rise in IL-6.

Ref: BJA 1996: 77; 569–570.

3.21 Osseous metastases due to prostate cancer **Answers: A C E**

The pain from boney metastases due to prostate cancer can be relieved by radiotherapy, orchidectomy or stilboestrol. Opioids and NSAIDs may also be of benefit.

3.22 Carotid sheath **Answers: A B C**

The carotid sheath contains the carotid artery, internal jugular vein and the vagus nerve.

3.23 One lung anaesthesia **Answers: A B C**

During one lung anaesthesia continued perfusion of the unventilated lung increases true shunt and venous admixture.This leads to hypoxia which, as it is true shunt, cannot be corrected by increasing the inspired oxygen entration. Hypoxia is normally minimised by compensatory HPV, but this may be abolished by the anaesthetic agents. Other ways of minimising hypoxia include the application of PEEP to the dependent lung, CPAP to the collapsed lung or using large tidal volumes.

3.24 Pulse oximeters **Answer: C**

Pulse oximeters do not cause burns, and although they do not read in real time they are nevertheless much faster than transcutaneous oxygen electrodes. They are inaccurate in the presence of both carboxy- and met-haemoglobin. As HbF and adult HbA have similar absorption spectra pulse oximeters are not inaccurate in the presence of HbF. Pigmented skin does not affect the accuracy of pulse oximeters.

3.25 Hyperkalaemia **Answers: A C**

Hyperkalaemia leads to a prolonged PR interval, flattened P waves, widened QRS complexes and tall peaked T waves. Hypokalaemia is associated with U waves; delta waves are seen in the Wolf-Parkinson-White syndrome.

3.26 Salicylate poisoning **Answers: D E**

It is salicylate poisoning that is associated with an early metabolic acidosis and hyperventilation. The main danger of paracetamol poisoning is liver damage. Normally 90% of paracetamol is conjugated by the liver with glucuronide or sulphate and excreted by the kidneys. A small amount is converted to a toxic metabolite which is normally then conjugated with glutathione and excreted by the kidneys. In overdose the glutathione is exhausted leaving the toxic metabolite free to cause centrilobular necrosis of the liver. Either oral methionine or intravenous acetylcysteine can be used as treatment up to 24 hours after the overdose to prevent the hepatic damage by the toxic metabolite. They act by replenishing the exhausted glutathione stores and mopping up the reactive metabolite.

3.27 Oliguria **Answers: B E**

Oliguria is the excretion of a urine volume too low for renal homeostatic mechanisms to maintain normal blood concentrations of waste products. The result is a rise in the plasma concentrations of urea, creatinine and potassium. In acute tubular necrosis (ATN) small amounts of poor quality urine are produced. Since the tubules fail to reabsorb sodium adequately it is found in high concentrations in the urine. The urine itself has a low osmolality and there is a failure to excrete urea, with a low urinary urea. The CVP rises as the kidneys fail to excrete water; ultimately this may lead to pulmonary oedema.

By comparison oliguria due to pre-renal failure is a physiological response to poor renal perfusion and leads to the production of small amounts of concentrated urine. As the kidneys are actually functioning normally the response is to conserve sodium, so the urinary sodium is

ADULT ADVANCED LIFE SUPPORT

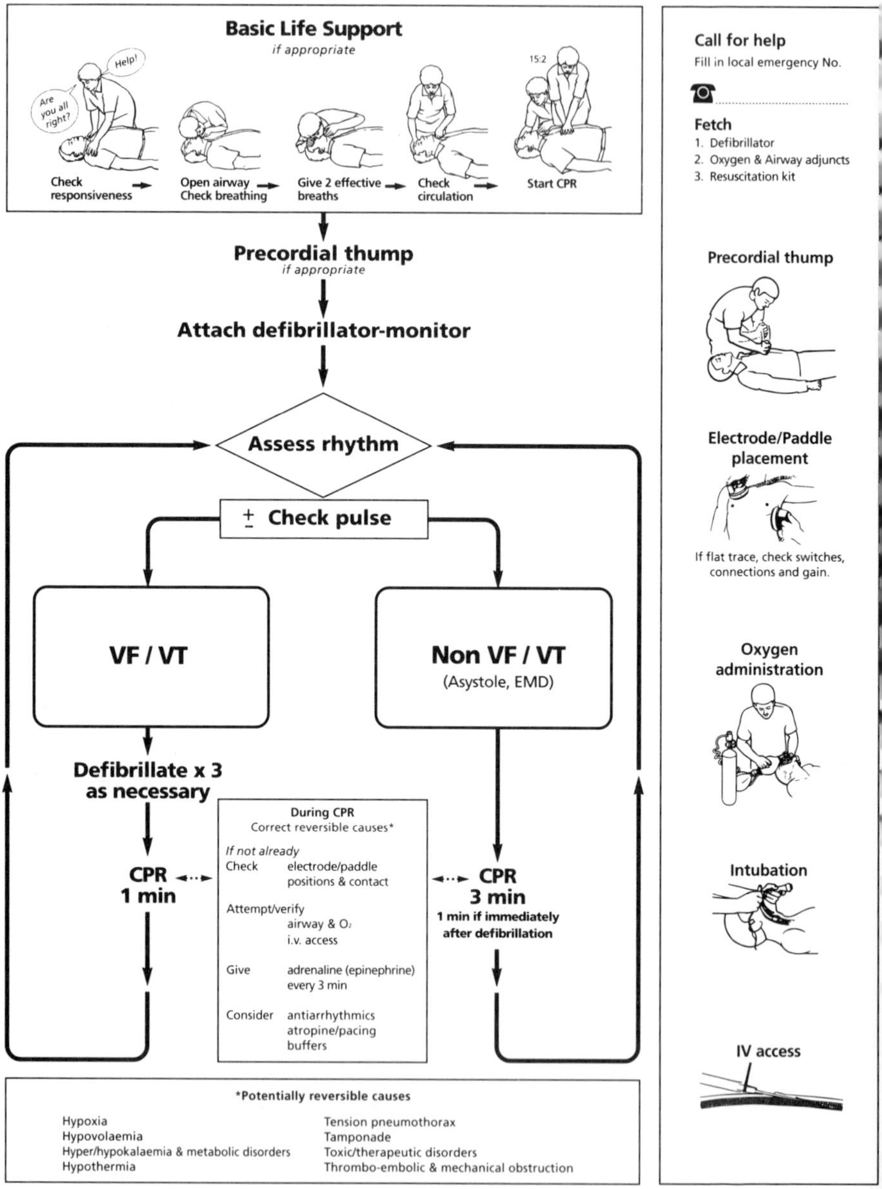

European Resuscitation Council in co-operation with Resuscitation Council (UK)

Available from
LAERDAL MEDICAL LTD.
Laerdal House, Orpington, Kent BR6 0HX
Tel. 01689 876634, Fax 01689 873800

low, while urea is appropriately excreted and the urinary urea is high. Most cases of pre-renal failure are due to hypovolaemia from dehydration or haemorrhage. Thus the CVP is low and the treatment is to give fluids and/or blood to expand the vascular volume and return renal perfusion to normal.This is clearly not appropriate management for ATN, and is why it is important to differentiate correctly between the two causes of oliguria.

3.28 Cardiac arrest **Answers: A C D E**

The chances of survival following cardiac arrest when the rhythm is VF decline exponentially with the time taken to defibrillation. If a VF arrest is witnessed, for example in a patient in CCU with ECG monitoring attached, then often a simple pre-cordial thump will restore sinus rhythm. Calcium is only indicated in cases of electro-mechanical dissociation (or PEA - pulseless electrical activity as it is now known) associated with hypocalcaemia or hyperkalaemia or the patient is on a calcium channel blocker. 8.4% sodium bicarbonate is a hyperosmolar solution. Its use is controversial as it may actually worsen intracellular acidosis. The latest ERC recommendations (as shown) are that bicarbonate should only be used if rescusitation is prolonged and where blood gases show an acidosis in the context of normocapnoea. Mannitol has been used to reduce cerebral oedema post arrest. Post arrest hyperglycaemia requires insulin as a high blood glucose is negatively inotropic.

3.29 Tetanus **Answers: A B C D**

Tetanus results from the actions of the exotoxin (tetanospasmin) of the bacillus *Clostridium tetani*. Tetanospasmin leads to generalised muscle rigidity and sympathetic overactivity. There may be respiratory compromise requiring ventilation. Human antitetanus antitoxin will neutralise exotoxin not yet fixed in the CNS. Active immunization with tetanus toxoid prevents the disease, but boosters are required every 10 years or on injury if the last booster was more than 5 years previously. The incubation period is 2–45 days.

3.30 Hypoxic mixture **Answers: A C D**

10% Oxygen is a hypoxic mixture. Hypoxia leads to central cyanosis and a reduced mixed venous oxygen content, as the tissues extract more oxygen to prevent tissue hypoxia. Organs such as heart, CNS and kidneys are highly susceptible to ischaemic damage due to their high oxygen consumption. Hypoxia will lead to myocardial depression with a fall in stroke volume and cardiac output. Anginal pain will occur if there is coronary atheroma.

3.31 Colloids **Answers: A D E**

The colloids are plasma expanders. The four main types are given below.

1. Gelatins (e.g. haemaccel, gelofusine)

They have a MW of 30–35,000 and an oncotic pressure similar to plasma. They do not cause renal failure or impair blood cross matching, but can cause allergic reactions. Haemaccel contains calcium and will cause citrated blood to clot if it comes into contact.

2. Dextrans (e.g. dextran 70)

The dextrans may cause renal failure, impair grouping and cross matching of blood and impair haemostasis by reducing factor 8 concentration and platelet adhesiveness.

3. Starches (e.g. hetastarch)

Hetastarch contains very large molecules of MW up to 450,000. Thus the plasma expansion is slightly greater than the volume of starch infused, and lasts in excess of 24 hours.The starches can impair renal function and impair haemostasis, by prolongation of the APTT, PT and bleeding time. They cause reduced levels of factor 8 and von Willebrand's factor. They are associated with a syndrome of intractable pruritus.

Ref: Anaesthesia & Analgesia 1997: 84; 206–212.
Ref: Br J Hosp Med 1995: 54; 155–159.

4. Human albumin

4.5% human albumin has a very similar oncotic presure to plasma, as the normal plasma albumin is about 45 g/l.

Ref: BMJ 1995: 310; 887–888.

3.32 Ritodrine **Answer: C**

Ritodrine is an agonist at beta-2 adrenoreceptors. It is used specifically to arrest premature labour. Like salbutamol, another beta-2 agonist, it produces tachycardia, peripheral vasodilatation and hypotension. Other side-effects include hypokalaemia and pulmonary oedema.

3.33 Drugs precipitating bronchospasm **Answers: A B C**

Aspirin and the NSAIDs may produce bronchospasm. Morphine may cause histamine release and therefore produce bronchospasm. Labetalol, like all beta blockers, can cause bronchoconstricton. All the volatile agents are bronchodilators, as is ketamine.

3.34 Wright's respirometer **Answers: D E**

The Wright's respirometer is used to measure inspired and expired lung volumes. It under-reads when the vanes are wet and at low tidal volumes.

3.35 Central venous pressure **Answers: A B C D**

The central venous pressure is a measure of right heart filling pressure (preload).The most accurate readings are obtained if the catheter tip lies in the lower superior vena cava or the right atrium. The classical a, c and v waves are transmitted from the right atrium to the internal jugular vein but are not seen in the axillary vein. With IPPV the normal physiological drop in CVP with inspiration is reversed as the intrathoracic pressure rises and blood is pushed out of the thoracic cavity.

3.36 Ionised calcium **Answers: A B C D E**

The total blood calcium consists of ionised (free) calcium and protein bound calcium. The ionised calcium is affected by pH and the serum albumin.The binding of calcium to albumin is pH dependent such that a rise in pH (alkalosis) leads to a reduction in the ionised fraction. As calcium is bound to albumin the serum calcium has to be adjusted by adding 0.2 mmol/l for every 10 g that the albumin is below 45 g/l.

3.37 Thiazides **Answers: A C E**

The thiazides may cause hyperglycaemia. All steroids including the OCP can impair glucose tolerance. Although the beta blockers can mask the autonomic response to hypoglycaemia they do not impair glucose tolerance.

3.38 Porphyric crisis **Answers: A B E**

The signs of a porphyric crisis include tachycardia, pyrexia, psychosis and the passing of urine which darkens on standing. Renal colic is not a symptom of porphyric crises but abdominal pain can occur.

3.39 Halothane **Answers: A C D E**

Halothane will absorb ultraviolet and infra-red radiation and will cause a change in the elasticity of silicone rubber. Halothane concentration can also be determined by a refractometer. Halothane has a MW of 197 daltons whereas the MW of nitrous oxide is 44 daltons.

Ref: Key topics in Anaesthesia by Craft and Upton 2nd edition, p 126–128.

3.40 Intraocular pressure (IOP) Answers: A E

Intraocular pressure (IOP) is raised by hypoxia, hypercarbia, hypertension and elevated venous pressure. Acetazolamide acts by inhibiting the enzyme carbonic anhydrase. The result is a reduced production of aqueous humour and a consequent reduction in intraocular pressure. Atropine, by causing mydriasis, improves aqueous drainage. While all the volatile agents and both propofol and thiopentone reduce IOP, suxamethonium causes an increase in IOP.

3.41 Suxamethonium Answers: A B E

Suxamethonium normally leads to an increase in serum potassium of 0.5–1.0 mmol/l. Certain patients can develop greater rises in potassium, predisposing to malignant ventricular arrythmias. Rhabdomyolysis from trauma produces hyperkalaemia. Blood contains a higher potassium than plasma; transfusion can cause hyperkalaemia. Intravenous bicarbonate and calcium gluconate are used to treat hyperkalaemia.

3.42 Nimodipine Answers: A C D

Nimodipine is a calcium channel blocking drug. It acts preferentially on cerebral arteries and is used specifically to prevent vasospasm and ischaemia following subarachnoid haemorrhage. Like all calcium antagonists it is a hypotensive agent. While diltiazem and verapamil enhance the effect of theophyllines, nimodipine has no effect.

3.43 Coeliac plexus block Answers: A B C D E

Coeliac plexus block is used to manage pain in conditions such as pancreatic cancer and chronic pancreatitis. Side-effects of the block include orthostatic hypotension, impotence and constriction of the sphincter of Oddi.

3.44 Reactions to intravenous dextrans Answers: A B C D

The incidence of allergic reactions to the dextrans is less than most of the colloids, except for human albumin. The incidence of anaphylactoid reactions is $< 0.1\%$.

3.45 Hyoscine Answers: B D

Hyoscine is marketed as a patch for motion sickness. Fentanyl is also available in a transdermal preparation for the treatment of malignant pain.

3.46 Propofol **Answers: B D**

Propofol is presented in a white aqueous emulsion containing 10% soyabean oil (intralipid), 1.2% purified egg phosphatide and 2.25% glycerol. It causes a drop in blood pressure of 15–25%, due to a reduction in cardiac output and peripheral vasodilatation. There is usually a reflex tachycardia. Propofol usually causes apnoea after induction and decreases the ventilatory response to hypercarbia. It reduces intraocular pressure and, bizarre though it sounds, may rarely cause green urine!

3.47 Bupivacaine **Answers: A B D**

Bupivacaine is an amide local anaesthetic. It is highly protein bound. All the local anaesthetic agents are safe in malignant hyperpyrexia. The main disadvantage of the agent is its cardiotoxicity, especially in pregnant women. There have been reports of it leading to refractory ventricular fibrillation in parturients and when used for intravenous regional anaesthesia (IVRA). It is thus no longer used for IVRA, where prilocaine is the agent of choice. In obstetric anaesthesia it may not be used in a concentration of more than 0.5%

3.48 Premature neonates **Answers: A B D E**

Premature neonates are more likely than term babies to suffer from hypothermia, hypocalcaemia and hypoglycaemia. They are often mildly jaundiced and are sensitive to the effects of the non-depolarising muscle relaxants.

3.49 Persistent vomiting **Answers: B D E**

Persistent vomiting leads to dehydration and other metabolic problems that must be corrected prior to surgery. In pyloric stenosis there is obstruction to gastric outlet and so the vomitus will be free of bile. Biliary atresia is seen more commonly in Down's syndrome.

3.50 Lignocaine **Answers: A C**

Lignocaine is the treatment of choice for ventricular ectopic beats during anaesthesia. Ischaemia, hypercarbia, electrolyte imbalance and a high level of circulating catecholamines predispose to the problem. The beta adrenoceptor blocking drugs may also prevent ventricular ectopics. Carotid sinus pressure and verapamil may be used in supraventricular tachycardia, although adenosine is now first-line therapy. Digoxin increases ventricular excitability and is not a treatment for ventricular ectopics. Its use is in atrial fibrillation, especially if associated heart failure is present.

3.51 Cardioversion **Answers: B E**

DC is used rather than AC for cardioversion. Sedation may be adequate rather than general anaesthesia. The shock should be at the start of the QRS complex. R on T may occur if the shock is not synchronised, resulting in VF.

3.52 Acid aspiration **Answers: A B D E**

Treatment of acid aspiration may involve bronchoscopy and bronchial lavage. Artificial ventilation may be required and steroids may be of some benefit; antibiotics are usually withheld unless there is evidence of infection.

3.53 Oxytocin **Answers: A C**

Oxytocin (syntocinon) and ergometrine are used to induce or augment labour and to minimise blood loss from the placental site. Oxytocin is produced endogenously in the posterior pituitary. It has actions similar to the other posterior pituitary hormone, ADH. Thus it causes fluid retention which can be severe enough to lead to water intoxication and convulsions. It causes peripheral vasodilatation with hypotension and reflex tachycardia. Oxytocin is very short acting. Ergometrine is a vasoconstrictor and causes hypertension and a high incidence of nausea and vomiting.

3.54 Agents to relax the uterus **Answers: A D E**

Thiopentone, halothane and the other volatile agents will all relax the uterus.Suxamethonium and the non-depolarising muscle relaxants act at the neuromuscular junction of striated muscle; they have no effect on the smooth muscle of the uterus. Ritodrine and salbutamol are beta 2 adrenergic receptor agonists and can be used to relax the uterus.

3.55 Cardiovascular changes in pregnancy **Answers: A C D**

The cardiovascular changes in pregnancy include an increase in heart rate and stroke volume and a fall in systemic vascular resistance. The result is that there is a fall in diastolic and mean blood pressure. Although total red cell mass increases there is a greater increase in plasma volume and hence a dilutional anaemia.

3.56 Anaphylactic reactions **Answers: B D E**

Anaphylactic reactions are type 1 hypersensitivity reactions, mediated by specific IgE antibodies. In a previously sensitised individual antigen and antibody bind to and then lead to the degranulation of mast cells and basophils. Release of histamine, serotonin and other cytokines leads to the clinical manifestations of urticaria, hypotension and bronchospasm. Anaphylactoid reactions are also the result of mast cell degranulation, but this is mediated directly by the drug, without involvement of IgE.

The most commonly implicated anaesthetic drugs include suxamethonium and some non-depolarising muscle relaxants, opioids, penicillins and NSAIDs. The colloids and latex rubber are important aetiologically to anaesthetists. Treatment must include adrenaline as a first-line drug. Its alpha agonist effect reverses vasodilatation and its beta agonist effect reverses bronchoconstriction and increases the force of myocardial contraction. Oxygen and plasma volume expansion are required.

Antihistamines and corticosteroids are useful second-line drugs. Salbutamol, aminophylline, isoflurane and ketamine may be used for refractory bronchospasm.

When investigating a reaction the serum mast cell tryptase is a sensitive and specific test for confirming that mast cell degranulation has occurred. Referral of the patient to an immunologist allows identification of the allergen by demonstrating specific IgE antibodies by either skin-prick test or radio-allergosorbent test (RAST).

A CSM Yellow card should be filled in and the patients GP informed. The patient should be fully informed and encouraged to carry an anaesthetic hazard card or wear a Medic-alert bracelet.

Ref: Suspected Anaphylactic Reactions Associated with Anaesthesia, 2nd Edition 1995. The Association of Anaesthetists of Great Britain and Ireland.

3.57 Supraclavicular brachial plexus block **Answers: A B C D E**
3.58 Axillary brachial plexus block **Answer: A**

There are three commonly used routes to block the brachial plexus: the axillary, interscalene and supraclavicular. The axillary route is probably the safest, while the supraclavicular is associated with a significant chance of pneumothorax. Other hazards of the supraclavicular route include subclavian artery puncture, and damage to the phrenic nerve, recurrent laryngeal and the cervical sympathetic trunk. The interscalene block is the most likely of the three routes to lead to either subarachnoid or extradural injection of local anaesthetic. The other main hazard with this route is injection into the vertebral artery.

3.59 Intercostal block **Answers: A B C**

With an intercostal block the local anaesthetic is deposited between the internal and innermost intercostal muscles, in the subcostal groove, where the neurovascular bundle lies. Injected local anaesthetic will spread both to the opposite side and up and down one or two segments. Bilateral blocks are contraindicated because of the risk of pneumothorax.

3.60 Caudal anaesthesia **Answers: B E**

The caudal space is the sacral continuation of the extradural space. As the dural sac ends at S2 it is possible to enter the subarachnoid space with a caudal injection. The needle used for the caudal should not be inserted beyond a depth of 2–3 mm once the sacrococcygeal membrane has been pierced. Although far less likely, puncture of the fetal head has been reported. A catheter technique can be used in the caudal canal.The failure rate for caudals is higher than for other types of epidurals and because of the larger volume of the caudal space a greater volume of local anaesthetic is required to produce a given block than would be necessary for a lumbar epidural.

3.61 Epidural test dose **Answers: B E**

An epidural test dose is used to detect inadvertent intravenous or subarachnoid injection. If a test dose is given intrathecally it produces a rapid, dense motor block in the legs. Intravenous injection may produce no effect, however. The patient sometimes complains of peri-oral paraesthesiae or light headedness. If adrenaline is added to the test dose then intravenous injection may produce a tachycardia. However since there are many causes of tachycardia this is not a very specific test. An epidural test dose will delay rather than hasten the onset of analgesia. It in no way prevents neurological complications, nor does it prevent tachyphylaxis which is simply a property of the local anaesthetic.

3.62 Ecstasy (MDMA) **Answers: A B C E**

It is estimated that Ecstasy or MDMA (3,4-methylenedioxymeth-amphetamine) may lead to about 50 deaths annually in the UK. Like other amphetamines its injection causes sympathetic stimulation with tachycardia, hypertension, myriasis and sweating. With profound sympathetic overactivity there may be hyperpyrexia, rhabdomyolysis, myoglobinuria and acute renal failure with DIC, convulsions, hyperkalaemia and metabolic acidosis, coma and death may supervene. In some deaths from MDMA water intoxication has caused death from acute cerebral oedema. There are many similarities with malignant hyperpyrexia and dantrolene is now used to treat MDMA intoxication.

Parkinsonism can result from ingestion of the 'designer drug' MPTP, which has a high degree of cytotoxicity for the substantia nigra.

3.63 Pacemakers affected by anaesthetic drugs **Answers: A D E**

Pacemakers may be affected by anaesthetic drugs, MRI scanners, shivering, diathermy and many other factors. Bipolar diathermy is safer than unipolar. MRI scanning is absolutely contraindicated in pacemaker patients. A magnet placed over a demand pacemaker will convert it to fixed rate mode.

3.64 Moffet's solution **Answers: A B C**

Moffet's solution contains 10% (100 mg/ml) cocaine. This is combined with adrenaline at a concentration of 0.1 mg/ml and 1% bicarbonate. The adrenaline intensifies the vasoconstrictor effect of the cocaine but increases the level of circulating catecholamines, predisposing to arrythmias. In combination with halothane and hypercarbia in, for example, a spontaneously ventilating patient, the result may be ventricular fibrillation. Moffet's is not used as analgesia. The safe maximum dose for cocaine when applied to the nasal mucosa is 1.5 mg/kg.

Ref: BMJ 1995: 311; 250–251.

3.65 Transplantation of the ureter in the colon **Answers: B D**

Transplantation of the ureter in the colon is the textbook example of a condition causing a hyperchloraemic acidosis. There is reabsorption of urinary urea by the colonic mucosa causing a rise in blood urea. There is hypokalaemia caused by the kidneys' attempts to retain bicarbonate in exchange for hydrogen and potassium ions.

3.66 Hypothermia **Answers: B D**

Hypothermia may occur in the elderly especially in winter if they collapse and are not discovered for some time. It may occur following a stroke, immersion in cold water, hypothyroidism, alcohol and drug intoxication. Myocardial depression, bradycardia with a J wave on the ECG, and arrthymias can occur below 28 °C. There is usually a metabolic acidosis and complications such as acute pancreatitis, hyperglycaemia, thrombocytopenia and DIC may occur.

3.67 Dopamine **Answers: A C D**

Dopamine is a naturallly occurring sympathetic amine; the endogenous precursor of noradrenaline. At low doses (2–4 mg/kg/min) dopamine stimulates dopamine 1 and 2 receptors, increasing renal blood flow, glomerular filtration rate and sodium excretion. Between 3 and 10 micrograms/kg/min dopamine stimulates beta-1-receptors causing positive inotrophy and chronotrophy. At doses above 10 mg/kg/min dopamine activates alpha receptors causing systemic vasoconstriction. There is currently much debate about the rationale for using low dose dopamine therapy in acute renal failure. Dopamine must be administred via a central line. It does not cross the blood-brain barrier.

Ref: BJA 1997: 78; 350–351.

3.68 Clonidine **Answers: A B C D**

Clonidine is a mixed alpha-2 and alpha-1 adrenergic agonist (alpha-2 : alpha-1 activity 200:1) It may be given orally, intravenously or epidurally. It produces hypotension by reducing central sympathetic outflow. The resulting unopposed parasympathetic vagal tone causes bradycardia. It is also a antisialogue, anxiolytic and sedative. Like the other alpha-2 agonists dexmedetomidine and medetomidine it reduces the MAC of volatile agents by up to 50%. Dexmedetomidine is used in veterinary anaesthetics as an induction agent and for maintanance of anaesthesia. It is even more selective for alpha-2 receptors than clonidine.

3.69 Post-partum headache **Answers: A B C D E**

Post-partum headache is most often non pathological (cephalgia fugax). Post dural puncture headache (PDPH) occurs in around 1% of mothers post spinal or epidural. The headache is typically aggravated by the upright posture and may be relieved by abdominal compression. Treatment may involve an epidural blood patch. Although rare, headache may be caused by subarachnoid haemorrhage or cortical vein thrombosis. Herpes simplex encephalitis may cause headache, convulsions and pyrexia. The CSF reveals a lymphocytosis and CT or MRI scanning show abnormalities in the temporal lobes. Treatment is with intravenous acyclovir.

3.70 Bier's block **Answer: C**

Because of its cardiotoxicity bupivacaine is contraindicated for a Bier's block. Prilocaine is the agent of choice; it may cause methaemoglobinaemia, not carboxyhaemoglobinaemia. Although a double tourniquet technique is often used it is not mandatory. The cuff should be inflated to 100 mmHg above systolic pressure and should not be deflated until at least 20 minutes after injection of local anaesthetic.

3.71 Caudal epidural block **Answers: A B C D**

The complications of caudal block include motor weakness, infection, delayed micturition and nausea and vomiting. Accidental intravenous or intraosseous injection can lead to systemic toxicity while dural puncture produces a high or even total spinal block.

3.72 Carbon monoxide poisoning **Answers: B C D**

Carbon monoxide (CO) has an affinity for haemoglobin of 250 times that of oxygen. The result is reduced oxygen carriage by haemoglobin and reduced oxygen delivery to the tissues. There is left shift of the oxyhaemoglobin dissociation curve. In addition there is histotoxic hypoxia as CO binds to and inhibits the enzymes of cellular respiration. The severity of the situation may be masked as the pulse oximeter overestimates the oxygen saturation, and the arterial oxygen tension is normal. Clinically CO poisoning produces tachycardia, decreased level of conciousness, convulsions and coma. There is often a metabolic (lactic) acidosis and hypokalaemia. The carboxyhaemoglobin (COHb) level must be measured to guide treatment. All patients should receive 100% oxygen. At a COHb level of > 40% hyperbaric oxygen therapy (HBO) should be considered. Since: $CaO_2 = Hb \times 1.34 + (PaO_2 \times 0.03)$ where CaO_2 is oxygen content, and $DO_2 = CaO_2 \times CO$ DO_2 is oxygen delivery and CO is cardiac output. With HBO therapy, at 300 kPa, the PaO_2 is sufficient, assuming a normal cardiac output, to meet average tissue oxygen requirements.

3.73 Infantile pyloric stenosis **Answers: A D**

Infantile pyloric stenosis causes projectile vomiting of gastric contents.The metabolic consequences are due to loss of HCl from the stomach; thus there is a metabolic alkalosis and hypochloraemia. The renal response to the resulting dehydration is to retain sodium and water in preferance to correcting the alkalosis. Thus there is paradoxical aciduria and renal loss of potassium causing hypokalaemia.This is a medical, but not a surgical, emergency. The priority is to correct the dehydration and acid-base disturbance prior to surgery.

3.74 Complex regional pain syndrome type 1 — Answers: A B C D

Complex regional pain syndrome type 1 (CRPS 1) was formerly known as reflex sympathetic dystrophy (RSD) or Sudeck's atrophy. CRPS II was formerly known as causalgia. CRPS type 1 involves sensory, motor and autonomic dysfunction. There may be osteoporosis and muscle atrophy in the affected limb. Allodynia (pain from normally inocuous stimuli),. hyperalgesia (normally painful stimuli cause severe pain), skin pallor, sweating and goose flesh can all be seen. Therapeutic sympathetic blocks (stellate ganglion blocks, for example) and guanethidine blocks are used to treat CRPS type 1.

3.75 Maternal mortality — Answers: A C D E

There were a total of 228 deaths, representing an overall mortality rate of 1 in 10,000. The commonest cause of death was thromboembolism (27.1%). Hypertensive disorders accounted for 15.5% of deaths. Haemorrhage accounted for 11.6%. Haemorrhage has been responsible, however, for more deaths than any other single cause since the CEMD began in 1952. Anaesthesia was directly responsible for 8 deaths and contributory in a further 6; hypoxia and airway obstruction being the problem in 5 of these deaths. There were 2 cases of fatal anaphylactic reactions to suxamethonium.

Ref: Report on Confidential Enquiries into Maternal Deaths in the United Kingdom, 1991–93. HMSO publications.

3.76 Measurement of oxygen in gases — Answer: E

The concentration of oxygen in a mixture of gases may be measured by mass spectrometry or a paramagnetic analyser. The Clark electrode or the fuel cell can measure the oxygen tension in blood or in a mixture of gases, respectively.

The pulse oximeter measures the saturation of haemoglobin with oxygen. The Severinghaus electrode measures the carbon dioxide tension in blood and the infrared analyser measures carbon dioxide tension in a mixture of gases.

The transcutaneous electrode measures the oxygen tension in blood *in vivo.*

3.77 Intrathecal opioids **Answers: A B D**

The four classic side-effects of intrathecal opioids such as fentanyl are pruritus, nausea and vomiting, urinary retention and respiratory depression. Piloerection (shivering) may occur. Respiratory depression may be severe enough to require naloxone. Pruritus is often mild but can be treated with a small dose of propofol or naloxone.

Ref: Can J Anaes 1995: 42; 891–903.

3.78 Magnetic resonance scanning **Answers: B C D**

Pacemakers are a contraindication to a patient entering the MRI scanner. All ferromagnetic objects must be outside the 50 G field. Monitoring may affect and be affected by MRI. A quench is due to a sudden leak of helium or nitrogen and can result in sudden asphyxia.

3.79 Bilirubin **Answers: D E**

Bilirubin is rendered water soluble by conjugation with glucuronide by the hepatocytes. Unconjugated bilirubin is bound to albumin but readily crosses the neonatal blood-brain barrier and can cause kernicterus. Phenobarbitone induces liver microsomal enzymes and enhances the conjugation process.

3.80 Nitrous oxide **Answer: B**

The pressure in a nitrous oxide cylinder is temperature dependent. At 20 °C it is 54 bar. Because nitrous oxide is present as a saturated vapour above a liquid the cylinder pressure only begins to fall once there is only vapour remaining. The critical temperature of nitrous oxide is 36.5 °C; Entonox has a critical temperature of -8 °C. The filling ratio of nitrous is 0.67. Although nitrous may cause megaloblastic changes in the bone marrow after prolonged exposure this is not due to vitamin B12 deficiency.

3.81 Stridor **Answers: A B C D**

Stridor is caused by glottic obstruction, due to oedema or a foreign body, and may be seen in croup, epiglottitis or tonsillitis. Bronchiolitis is caused by viral inflammation of the lower respiratory tract.

3.82 Minimum alveolar concentration (MAC) **Answers: A E**

MAC is reduced in the presence of nitrous oxide, premedication agents, myxoedema, with increasing age and atmospheric pressure. MAC is not affected by pregnancy or sex.

3.83 One lung anaesthesia **Answers: A B C D E**

One lung anaesthesia leads to a large shunt, since half the pulmonary blood flow is to unventilated lung.

The shunt equation is:

$$\frac{Qs}{Qt} = \frac{CcO_2 - CaO_2}{CcO_2 - C\bar{v}O_2}$$

Qs = Shunt fraction
Qt = Cardiac output
CcO_2 = Pulmonary vein oxygen content
$C\bar{v}O_2$ = Mixed venous oxygen content

CaO_2 (the oxygen content of arterial blood) is determined by the haematocrit and the oxygen tension of blood, PaO_2, since:

$$CaO_2 = Hb \times 1.34 + (PaO_2 \times 0.003)$$

Thus the shunt equation can be rewritten as:-

$$\frac{Qs}{Qt} = \frac{CcO_2 - [Hb + PaO_2]}{CcO_2 - C\bar{v}O_2}$$

Thus the PaO_2 depends on the haematocrit, cardiac output, mixed venous oxygen content and the amount of blood flow to the unventilated lung, the shunt fraction. The PaO_2 depends, of course, on the inspired oxygen tension.

3.84 Mapleson classification **Answers: A B C D E**

In 1954 Mapleson devised a classification for the breathing systems in use. They were labelled A–D; the Mapleson F breathing system was classified later. The A system is the Magill (or Lack coaxial version). It is the most efficient for spontaneous ventilation. The D system is the Bain, and is the most efficient for controlled ventilation. The E system is the Ayres T-piece and is the paediatric system used for patients of 20 kg or less. This system was modified by Jackson-Rees, who added an open-ended bag. This became the Mapleson F breathing system.

3.85 Intubation and ventilation of an elderly man **Answers: A B C E**

This man requires intubation and ventilation in view of his hypoxia and GCS of 6. The blood gases reveal a metabolic acidosis with an increased anion gap.

The anion gap formula is Na + K – Bic + Cl. The normal range is 9–14.

Causes of a metabolic acidosis with a raised anion gap include:

Lactic acidosis
Ketoacidosis

Renal failure
Salicylate and methanol poisoning
Rhabdomyolysis
Renal failure is excluded because of the normal K and urea, blood glucose. Salicylate and methanol intoxication are both possibilities.

3.86 Addison's disease **Answer: C**

Addison's disease is adrenocortical insufficiency. Lack of aldosterone and cortisol leads to loss of sodium and water and hence low blood pressure. There is hyperkalaemia, a mild metabolic acidosis and an inability to excrete a water load. It is treated with hydrocortisone and fludrocortisone.

3.87 Neonatal physiology **Answers: A B D**

In the neonate the stroke volume is relatively fixed and cardiac output increases are rate dependent.The liver is immature at birth and levels of vitamin K dependent clotting factors are low. The oxygen consumption of the neonate is approximately twice that of an adult. Circulating blood volume of the neonate is about 80–100 ml/kg.

3.88 Steroid treatment regimens **Answers: B C D E**

The current recommendations for steroid treatment are summarised in the table below:

Patients currently taking steroids	< 10 mg day $^{-1}$	Assume normal HPA response	Additional steroid cover not required
	> 10 mg day $^{-1}$	Minor surgery	25 mg hydrocortisone @ induction
		Moderate surgery	Usual pre-operative steroids + 25 mg hydrocortisone @ induction + 100 mg day $^{-1}$ for 24 h
		Major surgery	Usual pre-operative steroids + 25 mg hydrocortisone @ induction + 100 mg day $^{-1}$ for 72 h
	High dose immunosuppression	Give usual immunosuppressive doses during peri-operative period	
Patients stopped taking steroids	< 3 months	Treat as if on steroids	
	> 3 months	No peri-operative steroids necessary	

Ref: Anaesthesia 1998: 53; 1091–1104. Table reproduced by kind permission of Blackwell Science Ltd.

3.89 Oxygen therapy **Answers: A B C D**

While oxygen is clearly of benefit for all the other causes, retrolental fibroplasia is actually caused by oxygen!

3.90 Acute epiglottitis **Answer: C**

Acute epiglottitis is a bacterial infection most often caused by *Haemophilus influenzae* type B. Since the introduction of the HIB vaccine the incidence has fallen. While most cases occur in children it may occur in adults. Ampicillin or chloramphenicol are the antibiotics most often used. Intravenous access should wait until after a gentle inhalational induction; trying to secure venous access early may lead to total airway obstruction. Once the pyrexia has settled and there is an audible leak around the endotracheal tube, extubation is possible; usually after 24–48 hours.

PRACTICE EXAM 3: MODEL VIVA ANSWERS

Viva 1

Examiner 1

Summarise the case and the possible anaesthetic implications.
This is an elderly lady with severe rheumatoid disease and oesophageal reflux.
In view of her reflux she would, if a general anaesthetic was used, require a rapid sequence induction. However, in view of her rheumatoid disease affecting the cervical spine, intubation might be hazardous. A regional technique might therefore be the most appropriate anaesthetic.

Describe the findings on the cervical spine X-ray. What is the significance?
The X-rays reveal subluxation of the atlanto-axial joint. Normally there is no gap between the odontoid peg and the arch of the atlas. Subluxation is present when the distance between the atlas odontoid process in the lateral flexion view is > 3 mm in patients over 44 years of age or > 4 mm in younger patients.

The problem is that the odontoid peg, which is normally held in position by the strong transverse ligament of the atlas, encroaches on the spinal canal in flexion with the risk of spinal cord compression.

Therefore laryngoscopy must be undertaken with care in rheumatoid patients with evidence of cervical spine disease and atlanto-axial subluxation.

Other problems with the airway in rheumatoid arthritis include:
1) Temporomandibular joint dysfunction which may cause reduced mouth opening rendering intubation difficult.
2) Crico-arytenoid joint arthritis which may produce laryngeal obstruction.

Ref: BMJ 1993: 306; 79-80.
Ref: Canadian J.An. 1993: 40; 154-159.
Ref: Anaesthetics 1993: 48; 989-997.

How would you anaesthetise this lady?
I would opt for a regional technique. The options are:
i) epidural
ii) spinal
iii) combined spinal and epidural
iv) combined sciatic and femoral nerve blocks
v) intravenous regional anaesthesia of the lower limb.

The first three options are probably the most straightforward choices.

Examiner 2

What do you think the diagnosis is?
The findings of widely dilated pupils, tachycardia and convulsions in an unconscious patient who has taken some tablets strongly suggest an overdose of tricyclic anti-depressants.

The blood gases are typical. There is a marked metabolic acidosis (bicarbonate 11.4) and hypokalaemia.

The ECG shows bizarre QRS complexes with right bundle branch block and left posterior fascicular block (i.e. bifascicular block). Tricyclics have antichlolinergic effects which cause cardiac rhythm disturbances.

What is your management?
A B C
The airway is best secured by endotracheal intubation and artificial ventilation. She is likely to be hypovolaemic and will require intravenous fluids. Gastric lavage must be performed, samples of any tablets sent for analysis and activated charcoal instilled into the stomach to prevent further absorption of the drug.
Magnesium might be a useful anticonvulsant here and it may also act as an anti-arrhythmic.
The hypokalaemia should be corrected. The patient should be transferred to ITU.

What does the second ECG show?
What is your management?
This shows ventricular tachycardia. The management is according to ERC guidelines 1997:
1) Give precordial thump
2) Deliver 3 DC shocks as necessary

3) CPR for 1 minute
4) Give epinephrine every 3 minutes.

Consider bicarbonate if prolonged resuscitation.
Consider anti-arrthymics such as amiodarone, bretylium etc.

Viva 2

Examiner 1

What does the chest X-ray show?
What is the likely underlying diagnosis?
The PA chest X-ray shows a well circumscribed partly calcified mass at the upper left heart border. The lateral chest X-ray shows it to be an anterior mediastinal mass and in view of her history of medication for weakness this suggests that the mass is a thymoma and that the patient has myasthenia gravis.

What is myasthenia gravis?
What medications and other treatments are there for this condition?
Myasthenia gravis is an autoimmune disease in which there are antibodies to the post-synaptic acetylcholine receptor of the neuromuscular junction. It results in weakness mainly of proximal limb, facial and eye muscles. It is associated with other autoimmune conditions and patients may have a thymoma.

Management includes pharmacological treatment. Anticholinesterase drugs such as pyridostigmine, increase the level of acetylcholine at the neuromuscular junction. An alternative approach is to use immunosuppressive agents such as azathioprine or steroids. Non-pharmacological treatments include plasmapheresis and thymectomy.

What are the anaesthetic implications of myasthenia gravis?
The main consideration is the response of these patients to muscle relaxants. They require a much smaller dose of non-depolarising muscle relaxant. By contrast they are resistant to suxamethonium and exhibit unusual and sometimes prolonged blocks.

Examiner 2

Here is a CT scan of the brain of a young man who presented to A&E having been knocked unconscious playing rugby. He was initially lucid after regaining consciousness but then lapsed into coma.

What does the scan show?
The CT scan shows a hypodense area in the right cerebral hemisphere. There is evidence of midline shift and compression of the lateral ventricle. The biconvexity of the lesion suggests it is an extradural haematoma. (The other CT scan, for comparison, shows the typical concavo-convex shape of a subdural haematoma.)

Describe your initial management of this man in A&E.
According to the ATLS guidelines my priorities are:

A airway (with cervical spine control)
B breathing
C circulation (with haemorrhage control)
D dysfunction (neurological assessment, including GCS)
E exposure (to identify all injuries).

The aim is to prevent secondary brain damage by preventing hypoxia and hypotension and then once stabilised to refer the patient to the neurological team for evacuation of the haematoma.
Indications for immediate endotracheal intubation and ventilation after head injury are:

1. GCS ≤ 8
2. Ventilatory insufficiency
   a) $PaO_2 < 9$ kPa on air or < 13 kPa with O_2
   b) $PaCO_2 > 6$ kPa
3. Loss of protective laryngeal reflexes
4. Respiratory arrythmia
5. Spontaneous hyperventilation causing $PaCO_2 < 3.5$ kPa

Intubation must be carried out with cervical spine control in case of a coexisting cervical spine injury. A rapid sequence induction should be performed. Thiopentone is the induction agent of choice as it is also an anticonvulsant and reduces cerebral metabolism. A short-acting opioid will reduce the pressor response to laryngoscopy and intubation.
Two large bore (14 G) IV cannulae should be inserted and appropriate fluids

given as necessary.
Since CPP = MAP- ICP; in this patient a MAP of 90 mmHg should be maintained. Ideally intracranial pressure monitoring should be instigated.
There should be a full neurological assessment including the GCS and full exposure of the patient to check for other injuries.
An arterial line to monitor blood pressure and blood gases would be useful.
The PaO_2 should be kept above 13 kPa and the $PaCO_2$ 4-4.5 kPa.
Pulse oximetry, ECG, end tidal CO_2 and urine output should be monitored, as well as regular neurological observations and fluid balance. The patient must be kept sedated and pain free.

Ref: **BMJ 1993: 307; 547-552**
Ref: **Recommendations for the transfer of patients with acute head injuries to neurosurgical units by the Neuroanaesthetic Society of Great Britain and Ireland and the Association of Anaesthetists of Great Britain and Ireland. Dec 1996.**

MCQ REVISION INDEX

The number against each item refers to the examination and question number.